FIND THIS BOOK WILL PROVIDE YOU WITH INVALUABLE INSIGHT.

GOD BLESS YOU ALWAYS!

Mary Bayer

9/15/16

I PROMISE
I'LL PAY ATTENTION

I PROMISE
I'LL PAY ATTENTION

LIVING WITH A SEEMINGLY INVISIBLE, PROGRESSIVELY DEBILITATING DISEASE

GARY BEYER

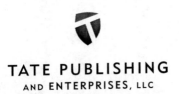

TATE PUBLISHING
AND ENTERPRISES, LLC

Published by Tate Publishing & Enterprises, LLC
127 E. Trade Center Terrace | Mustang, Oklahoma 73064 USA
1.888.361.9473 | www.tatepublishing.com

Tate Publishing is committed to excellence in the publishing industry. The company reflects the philosophy established by the founders, based on Psalm 68:11,
"The Lord gave the word and great was the company of those who published it."

Published in the United States of America

ISBN: 978-1-68301-456-0
1. Medical / Osteopathy
2. Medical / Long-Term Care
16.05.17

Contents

This book is humbly dedicated to my awesome wife and caregiver, Julie...as well as to the numerous other caregivers out there who so selflessly honor the lives of those they love, respect, and/or immeasurably care for. Their all-important roles can be overlooked, underestimated, misinterpreted, and misunderstood by others who interact with the sufferer. More commonly, this is not the case with regard to the sufferers themselves.

I am truly grateful to be blessed with such a treasure. It's the type of gift that only God can arrange. We move forward together, facing our anticipated challenges with forthright determination and courage. There is no running from them, there is no hiding from them, but thanks to the tremendous assistance of our caregivers, we continue to fight the good fight.

God bless you, my beloved Julie, and thank you again!

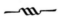

Special acknowledgement to Loralee L. Olson-Arcand of Word Services Unlimited (www.wordservicesunlimited.com) for the extensive preliminary layout work and print-ready work she did for me in conjunction with the development of this book, to John Steshetz of Proforma Printxx (www.proforma.com/printxx) for his strong encouragement and support in this effort.

Also, my good friend, photographer Rick Ramirez (owner of Look! That's My Kid Photography)—www.lookthatsmykid.com, who actually suggested and took the front photo of this book and also designed its front and back covers.

Especially to my wife Julie for her considerable guidance, expertise and support throughout this spiritually-driven effort and also for being my primary editor (she was a highly respected high school English teacher for 34 1/2 years).

The Days

The days all seem different to me now
They have for quite some time
They often bring with them changes
Which seem aimed directly at my mind

Many times the changes are subtle
While at other times they are just simply strange
Their impact can become quite dramatic
With less-refined intentions that yet seem prearranged

When I take the time to think about it
My perspectives have been substantially altered
As I acknowledge I'm fighting a formidable daily battle
Through which I've noticeably weakened and also
faltered

I've found this disease to be progressively relentless
And it's always there to be faced
There is no disputing, running or hiding
But I'm doing my best to stay in this most treasured race

I'm determined to not let its challenges overwhelm me
As I attempt to effectively deal with its various curves
The associated obstacles are steadily increasing
Causing the ongoing taxing of my nerves

What once seemed to be less relevant
Now seems to linger on and even disturbingly foretell
But, I still live each day with encouragement and hope
As my faith and beliefs will not be dispelled

Despite the days seeming different to me now
An important fact definitely still remains
I approach each one of them with refined vigor
Doing my best to cope with any consequential strains

I live in affirmed reality
But, I temper it with grit
A veil of gloom and disparity
Just can't be allowed to fit
(Gary Beyer [11/14/15])

Introduction

PEOPLE WHO HAVE gotten to know me would tell you that I am typically an upbeat person. The glass is usually half-full. My sincerest objective is to be happy. This was my answer to a question asked by my girlfriend (who was to become my wife). Now, this sounds pretty basic. I believe it's truly anything but that. Various complexities come into our lives. Some are self-imposed, while others are not. We can accomplish difficult tasks, achieve rewarding goals, and regularly satisfy our own, as well as others, expectations of us...but are we happy?

I am very happy. I am also extremely blessed and doing my best to live effectively with a progressively debilitating muscle disease that is seemingly invisible to most people.

I've always been a highly self-motivated person who was driven to succeed in mostly anything I've consciously attempted. I've been the most happy since I met Julie. By the middle of 2010, it was becoming more and more evident that the muscle condition I had was quite formidable. This was compounded by the fact that I was also experiencing some highly troublesome vision-related issues. I was pretty down, and most people around me didn't know it, not even the people who knew me well. The only one who detected it was Julie. I tried to hide it because I didn't want to further burden her with my emotional issues…she was far too busy with her own demanding job.

Back then, I was regularly sleeping in a recliner because it was easier for me and less disruptive for Julie. It had become clear that the ramifications from my uncontrollable, health-related issues were significantly overtaking our lives, not just mine. I've always believed in the power of prayer, but I found myself consistently adding a couple of additional sentences every night. I was asking God to help me figure this out.

These two sentences were: "Dear God, please give me some indications of what I should be doing. *I promise I'll pay attention.*"

Since April of 2012, I've been consistently sleeping in a hydraulic lift chair. One early morning in late July of 2013, I woke up and sat up straight in the chair. I'll never forget this. It's like it was yesterday. The strongest and clearest thought ran through my mind. I was given the divine inspiration to pursue writing a book. The definitive title came to me in a matter of just two to three seconds thereafter… Honestly! It needed to be entitled, *You Must Answer This.* When my wife came down from the upstairs bedroom, I was still sitting straight up in the lift chair. She asked me if I was all right. She wondered if I had fallen. I likely had a smile on my face when I told her I was okay, but that I was going to pursue the writing of a book and that it would be entitled, *You Must Answer This*. She understood what this phrase was all about. What was she supposed to say to me at this time of the morning? "Good luck," "That's fine," "Whatever." About two weeks later on August 11th, I woke up, got my bearings, and determinably headed over to the higher desk chair in front of the first-floor computer to begin writing the outline for this book. I finished writing it just before our twenty-fifth wedding anniversary on October 1st, 2013. I found myself spiritually driven to write it and share its various compelling true stories with others. As I was getting closer to that date, I found myself believing I may be able to finish writing it by then. She didn't expect it, I had kept this as a surprise. After giving her an anniversary card at a supper club that evening, I presented her with a second envelope. Inside was a letter which expressed the dedication of this book to Julie. Quietly some tears came down her face. She said, "This is worth more to me than a million dollars." I told her, "I know it is…it's worth a lot to me too."

We need to learn to cherish all the wonderful things that are in our lives…many of which are around us every day. They may seem to be simple in nature, minimal in scope, modest in appearance, and comparatively abundant, but they shouldn't be taken for granted.

I recently awoke to a similar divine indication as I did prior to starting my first book. The direct result of this is *I Promise I'll Pay Attention*. I'm very proud of it, and I hope that you enjoy reading it. I know why this one came about, just like I do the first. The Holy Spirit's moved me and continues to move me in resoundingly inspirational ways. All glory be to God.

Be proactive and engaged in your life.
Don't let life just happen to you.

—Gary Beyer

You Look Good

REMEMBER THAT CAUTIONING statement we've probably all been given at one time or another of..."looks can be deceiving". We've, likely, found out at times that "no truer words were ever spoken". You can't tell a book by its cover.

We may have had a *crush* on someone we found attractive, only to find out that either you had nothing in common with that person or you were able to detect some specific behavioral traits you were incompatible with. How about the visually impressive car that had performance-related issues?

Unless we're around somebody long enough, we may not be able to identify any of the troublesome things that they're dealing with in their life. Oftentimes, for various reasons, we attempt to keep some of these things to ourselves. Many people are dealing with numerous issues every day. Some may be quite major, some are decisively minor, and some are just nagging and uncontrollable. Regardless, we may or may not detect signs of disruption or reasons for concern.

A person's physical posturing is also something we commonly use to base some of our opinions on. We've also likely found how inaccurate this can be. How about the person you encounter who seemingly "has it all together"? You may find out that this was all just smoke and mirrors.

Growing up, we're told to be ourselves. Physical appearance is part of the package we present to others. You've probably heard the phrase "clothes don't make the man," but a clean-looking, complementary pieced selection of clothes goes a long way toward giving a good impression. How about this one, "you can dress them up, but you can't take them anywhere." These phrases came about for a reason.

I have found that people seem to equate looking good with doing good. I consistently and quickly receive this comment from people I encounter "that know" I was diagnosed with a muscle disease: "You look good." There is typically no probing as to how I might be doing. My common answer of thank-you seems to be more than enough for them to quickly move on with any conversation. I'm not a complainer by nature, but it sure would be nice sometimes if that same person would take a short period of time to genuinely find out how I was actually doing. I'm not going to take this opportunity to go into a blow-by-blow detail of all the symptoms I'm regularly experiencing, but just the detection of some genuine interest would sure be appreciated.

Many people are uncomfortable probing how their friends and acquaintances are doing if they know that they are dealing with some specific troublesome matter(s) or health-related issue(s). However, I also believe it's a type of cop out and irresponsible behavior when their level of relationship with that other person should also consciously tell them that this person deserves that consideration. The excuse is: "I don't want to stick my nose where it doesn't belong." In reality, it likely does belong if you're a compassionate and considerate friend or longer-term acquaintance. If circumstances or conditions are such that the person isn't open to your well-meaning probing, they will let you know. There are times, like at funerals, when we find ourselves not knowing what to say, but we make the conscious effort(s) to let the impacted family members and close friends know that we care.

Specific signs and symptoms are associated with most types of diseases and conditions. With untreatable, progressive diseases, some of the defined signs occur at different times, and the symptoms are more visible to others when they're able to spend more time around the sufferer. As time moves on, the by-products of the progressions become more obvious to others. The visual component of most symptoms is what predominantly determines how their impact is perceived by others.

It's unfortunate because this factor can inappropriately minimize the impact of the symptoms that are being experienced by the sufferer. Looks can definitely be deceiving.

I was diagnosed with an inflammatory muscle disease known as inclusion body myositis in January of 2008. It is an asymmetric condition, meaning some symptoms are inconsistent in their degree of severity on each side of the body. It manifests itself in different ways. For example, my right leg is definitely stronger and more stable than my left. I always need to lead with it when walking or trying to go up a step. Yet I can pick my left leg up significantly higher than I can my right. Getting up to a standing position from a normal height, seated position (without considerable help from others) has become next to impossible for me at this stage. It has reached a point where I consciously remain standing in environments where I have no possible elevated option. I have consistent pain in the same muscle area (near the shoulder joints) of both upper arms when I attempt to raise my arms above my head. This pain shows itself when I engage the associated muscles which trigger this process. I've also detected some noticeable muscle-contraction...as the length of my reach from either arm has clearly lessened. The prominence of muscle-wasting is undeniable if I'm wearing a short-sleeved shirt.

Signs Associated With Inclusion Body Myositis:

Frequent falling episodes

Trouble climbing stairs or standing from a seated position

A foot that seems to drop when walking, causing tripping

Weakened hand grip

Difficulty swallowing

Symptoms Associated with Inclusion Body Myositis:[1]

Weakened or noticeable shrinking of quadriceps (main muscle of the thighs) causing falls

Weakness in the forearm muscles

Weakness of muscles below the knees causing the foot to drop and toes to catch when walking

Weakness of flexor muscles of the fingers (used for gripping)

Weakness of throat muscles causing trouble swallowing (dysphagia) and possibly choking

Pain or discomfort as muscles weaken

In the past, there were times when I saw people parking in handicap-assigned spaces, and I would question whether their handicap warranted such special treatment. They would get out of their vehicle and seem to be fine when walking toward their destination. That word "assume" comes in to play again. I'd effectively assume that I was able

---

1   http://www.facebook.com/groups/7950401889/
     (Inclusion Body Myositis-open group)

to determine whether they were "sufficiently handicapped" or not by just looking at them for awhile.

Well, my friends, we are all responsible for our interpretations of things. Limited information, incorrect information, and a tendency to pass hurried judgments regularly preclude our assumptions. The various diseases and disruptive conditions steadily impacting many people's lives are often at least somewhat invisible to others; if not even totally invisible. As a responsible friend of someone else that you know is dealing with some difficult things, please don't be disinclined to (respectfully) probe once in awhile...they'll likely appreciate it very much.

> When you're living with a progressively debilitative condition you find yourself becoming more and more a prisoner of your own body.
>
> —Gary Beyer

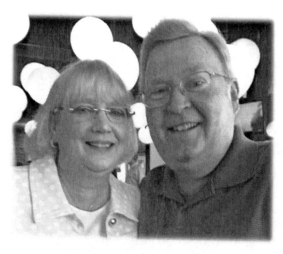

Julie and Gary in April of 2015

What Does the Term Rare Mean To You?

I CONSCIOUSLY CHOSE to use the designation of "term" rather than "word." This is because term seems more appropriate for distinguishing its potentially disturbing nature. The likelihood of encountering something "rare" in my life would surely be infrequent (if at all) and extremely atypical (if not special).

What I definitely didn't expect is that this term was to become so personally applicable in my life. For me, its mere mention brings thoughts of a wolf in sheep's clothing.

My father was forty-seven when I was born and my mother was forty-one. This was certainly not rare... albeit atypical. Like with most people there were some things encountered over the years that seemed quite unique at the time, but to classify them as rare would be too strong. Sure, there were also a number of infrequent, as well as, unusual things experienced, but they weren't worthy of being categorized as rare.

I was twenty-five in the early spring of 1979 when I was involved in a late-night collision with a sand truck, traveling in the opposite lane, carrying twenty-six tons of sand. This definitely fits my perception of the term rare above when it's combined with the fact that thanks to the grace of God, I was able to appreciably survive this major collision without any paralysis or associated disability.

By the time I reached the age of fifty, I had become sufficiently weary from my long-time exposure to the corporate world, thankful to be married to a wonderful woman, and was very blessed to be where I was in my life, both physically and mentally. I had definitely not burned out, but rather was thankfully in the process of becoming reinvigorated by a major change in careers. I had switched from being a corporate accountant to being a small business owner. I was proud of what I stood for, driven by some new challenges and, most importantly, was truly happy.

I loved what I was doing, but in the next few years something was definitely changing in my body. I had no idea what it was, but I was becoming noticeably weaker and my strength was declining. It seemed like "getting older" was catching up with me. What else could it be? There was really no pain or other side affects at that time.

In December of 2007, I made a doctor's appointment for a different reason. Even though the symptoms identified were more and more evident, at this point, I would not have made an appointment for these reasons. When I brought these other symptoms up near the very end of my visit with the physician's assistant, she thankfully took heed of them.

The results of a neuromuscular EMG precluded the recommendation for a thigh muscle biopsy in January of 2008. The Friday afternoon diagnostic telephone call from a neuromuscular specialist in Madison, Wisconsin, confirmed our worst fears. I was told that I had inclusion body myositis or IBM. This rare type of inflammatory muscle disease is considered an "orphan disease." Wikipedia references a study from 2008 whereby "the authors found that the current prevalence was 14.9 per million in the overall population, with a prevalence of 51.3 per million population in people over fifty years of age.²"

In mid-2010, I started experiencing vertical double vision. Later that year, I was diagnosed with diplopia and became a candidate for eye muscle-related strabismus surgery. Thankfully, the incorporation of prism-based corrective lenses have been able to successfully offset the

---

2   Needham M, Corbett A, Day T, Christiansen F, Fabian V, Mastaglia FL. (2008). "Dysphagia in inclusion body myositis: clinical features, management, and clinical outcome." J Clin Neurosci. 15 (12): 1350–3. Doi:10.1016/j.jocn.2008.01.011. PMID 18815046.

extremely disruptive impact of this condition without the need for this relatively inexact type of surgery. In late 2011, I needed to have cataract removal surgery done on each of my eyes. Then after a weekend (middle of the night) wake-up experience in early November of 2012, I clearly detected a jagged, half-moon-like figure appearing in my left eye. Fast-forward just a couple days, and I'm sitting in front of an eye surgeon being told that I have a retinal detachment in both of my eyes. He proceeded to tell me that it was extremely rare to have two eye detachments at the same time. In no uncertain terms, he also made it clear that I was about to go blind in each of my eyes. The next afternoon, I'm having emergency surgery on my left eye (by this surgeon) at a hospital in Green Bay. Next day, emergency surgery on the right eye would follow only a few weeks thereafter.

The formal definition of rare is "something that exists in limited quantities, that is unusually good, or meat that is not cooked until it is well done."[3]

It's important for us to recognize that words can connote different things to different people. We also need to realize that a person's perception of the same word can become significantly altered over time. Our interpretations are heavily influenced by our respective experiences and environment. We may or may not even realize it.

---

3   http://www.yourdictionary.com/rare

Rare can readily become a misused noun or an inappropriately used adjective, but I'll tell you what, with regard to myself, it has definitely become a term that brings with it some very uncomfortable and disconcerting feelings.

> I believe that God never gives us more
> than we can handle, but there are times
> when we're not as confident that we're up
> to the challenge(s) we are faced with.
>
> —Gary Beyer

The Unrelenting Daily Reality

WE ARE EACH faced with different health-related challenges during the course of our lives. Many are directly or indirectly the result of our own behavior and decision-making. A number of them are most impactful during a relatively short time frame and may involve some type of surgery in order to move beyond. There are often specific behavioral changes involved and potential therapy with an expected recovery period. We try to identify "the light at the end of the tunnel" that is associated with any projected recovery period. Normally, a defined care program is introduced to help us with the handling of certain types of health challenges. Recommended treatment typically includes specific medication along with follow up checkups and the input of various care professionals. Other health issues are attributable to our aging process or possibly environmentally related causes and care protocol is much less specific.

Identifying a recovery period is not possible when dealing with an untreatable, progressively deteriorating, chronic disease or condition. The unrelenting daily reality that needs to be faced (and consistently coped with) by both the sufferer and the caregiver is that this is just not the case. You can't allow yourself to get caught up in attempting to identify a time frame of recovery. In personally dealing with this type of condition, I've found it best to be as adaptive as possible and to address challenges a day at a time with a positive spin being a regular part of the process.

There is an ebb and flow which commonly exists during the time frames when our health challenges are being met. We find ourselves fortunate when a recovery process is steady, short, and easily defined. The sufferer wakes up each day and can detect for themselves that progress is definitely taking place. This especially helps in longer-term recoveries because a sense of comfort is derived from the belief that "relatively soon" we'll be better.

We've all had viruses like the common cold and flu. As the virus moves through its various phases, we find ourselves feeling different degrees of miserable. Headaches, disruptive running noses, and persistent coughing episodes make us feel like we should be on a short-term disabled list. How about the body aches and pains and related fatigue? We also know that we're not the most pleasant person to be around at such times. The severity of such viruses are minimized, but they take their toll on us, don't they? We always recognize, however, that this too will pass before very long.

As we get older, we find that many of the various exertions that we took for granted when we were younger now bring with them some form of lingering side effects. Reaching up to cut a few tree branches (and, of course, picking them up) also means that we'll realize unexpected muscle soreness for a few days. Washing your car becomes a much-bigger project than it once was. Did anyone else notice that the time frames associated with lingering side effects get seemingly longer too?

Pursuing relatively small, manageable home projects usually makes us feel good and gives us a nice sense of accomplishment. There comes a time though when many of these projects become more appropriately taken on by someone else. Our pride gives way to common sense and practicality. The "I can do it" mentality changes to "it's probably best if I don't try to do it myself."

I was always somewhat of a "putterer." I enjoyed identifying different projects that I believed I could successfully tackle. I wouldn't call myself a handyman, because I was never so inclined…nor was I mechanically oriented. Being an accountant, my skills were in analysis and problem-solving. The nice diversion I gained from puttering was a pleasant offset to the stresses I experienced in the corporate world.

Most of the challenges we encounter in our lives are of a definitive nature with regard to their resolution. The challenge is first recognized, an approach or plan of attack is identified, and then a time frame of completion is anticipated. It's normal for us to try to define resolutions to our challenges. Our health challenges can be explained in a similar fashion.

Since being diagnosed with inclusion body myositis in January of 2008, I've been consistently told that this remains a progressively, debilitating disease for which there is no recognized cure or treatment. I thankfully wake up every day with a positive mind-set. Nonetheless, the highly impactful presence of this condition is readily detectable. It is steadily progressing. It is unrelenting and if you let it, it will play with your mind because there are more and more things that I'm having significant difficulty doing. Many of these things I would classify as very basic activities.

I've found that it's now best to regularly err on the side of caution in what's become a revised approach to living our lives. I need to stay in tune with what my body is telling me and effectively communicate the implications to Julie. Like it is with many of you, the constraints that we're dealing with are very real. There's no accompanying intention of becoming recluses, but discretion is clearly the better part of valor. There also is no intent to offend anyone when I/we choose to turn down various invites that we would have otherwise readily accepted in the past.

The reminder of this condition is there for me each and every morning, but I quickly focus on two other reminders: my unrelenting faith in God and the incredible blessing I have in my wife, Julie.

LIFE ISN'T ABOUT
WAITING FOR THE
STORM TO PASS.
IT'S ABOUT LEARNING
HOW TO DANCE
IN THE RAIN...
-VIVIAN
GREENE

An Orphan Disease

DESCRIPTIVE ADJECTIVES ARE generally self-explanatory when accompanying a noun. They normally add a distinctive classification to it. Some are more descriptively effective than others like: torn muscle, blurred vision, and pounding headache. Then there are those combinations like: foreign-exchange student, love song, French poodle, and all-season tires that readily clarify a type of thing. How about this one... orphan disease. What is an *orphan disease* and why is this classification used for certain types of diseases?

> A rare disease, also referred to as an orphan disease, is any disease that affects a small percentage of the population. Most rare diseases are genetic, and thus are present throughout the person's entire life, even if symptoms do not immediately appear. [...][4]

---

4   "Rare Diseases." Siope.Eu. 2009-06-09. Retrieved 2012-09-24.

No single cutoff number has been agreed upon for which a disease is considered rare.

A disease may be considered rare in one part of the world, or in a particular group of people, but still be common in another.

There is no single, widely accepted definition for rare diseases. Some definitions rely solely on the number of people living with a disease, and other definitions include other factors, such as the existence of adequate treatments or the severity of the disease. In the United States, the Rare Diseases Act of 2002 defines rare disease strictly according to prevalence, specifically "any disease or condition that affects less than 200,000 people in the United States,"[5] or about 1 in 1,500 people. This definition is essentially like that of the Orphan Drug Act of 1983, a federal law that was written to encourage research into rare diseases and possible cures. In Japan, the legal definition of a rare disease is one that affects fewer than 50,000 patients in Japan, or about 1 in 2,500 people.[6] However, the European Commission on Public Health defines rare diseases as "life-threatening or chronically debilitating diseases which are of such low prevalence that special combined efforts are needed to address them."[7] The term low prevalence is later defined as

---

5   Rare Disease Act of 2002

6   Rare diseases: what are we talking about?

7   "Useful Information on Rare Diseases from an EU Perspective." European Commission. Retrieved 19 May 2009.

generally meaning fewer than 1 in 2,000 people. Diseases that are statistically rare, but not also life-threatening, chronically debilitating, or inadequately treated, are excluded from their definition. The definitions used in the medical literature and by national health plans are similarly divided, with definitions ranging from 1/1,000 to 1/200,000.[3]

Because of definitions that include reference to treatment availability, a lack of resources, and severity of the disease, the term *orphan disease* is used as a synonym for rare disease.[3] However, in the United States and the European Union, *"orphan diseases"* have a distinct legal meaning. The orphan drug movement began in the United States.[3] The United States' Orphan Drug Act includes both rare diseases and any non-rare diseases "for which there is no reasonable expectation that the cost of developing and making available in the United States a drug for such disease or condition will [be] recovered from sales in the United States of such drug" as *orphan diseases.*[8] The European Organization for Rare Diseases (EURORDIS) also includes both rare diseases and neglected diseases into a larger category of *"orphan diseases."*[9]

(Wikipedia)

---

8   Orphan Drug Act §526(a)(2)
9   "Rare Diseases: Understanding This Public Health Priority." European Organisation for Rare Diseases (EURORDIS). November 2005. Retrieved 16 May 2009.

Orphan Disease a disease for which no treatment has been developed because of its rarity (affecting no more than 200,000 persons in the U.S.).

(www.medilexicon.com/medicaldictionary. php)

Orphan disease: A disease that has not been adopted by the pharmaceutical industry because it provides little financial incentive for the private sector to make and market new medications to treat or prevent it. An orphan disease may be a rare disease (according to US criteria, a disease that affects fewer than 200,000 people) or a common disease that has been ignored (such as tuberculosis, cholera, typhoid, and malaria) because it is far more prevalent in developing countries than in the developed world.

(Medicinenet.com [Last Editorial Review: 3/19/ 2012])

5

Would You Prefer a Booth or a Table?

THE WORLD IS full of fundamental expectations. We learn to have such expectations of both ourselves and others. They have these expectations of us as well. Their basis is usually centered around some activity, response, or task. We expect to get out of bed every morning, get dressed and undressed, eat three meals a day, and go to bed every night. We're expected to attend school, get good grades, and find a job that is worthy of our time. We expect others to be kind, treat us with respect, and include us in various things. All of these things are *taken for granted*.

Then there are anticipations. We anticipate watching a particular television show, going to a specific restaurant, eating a well-cooked steak from your grill, being at a particular music or sporting event, celebrating a birthday, and enjoying time with family and friends. There are times when the excitement associated with the anticipation is almost as enjoyable as the *inevitable* event or activity.

———————

I grew up in a home which had radiant heat in the floors. It was so nice sitting or lying on the floor because it felt so good on my body. I thought nothing of being able to do this whenever I wanted to.

Later on, my parents added a second floor to this home. The addition included a really cool spiral stairway. I loved regularly going up and down it. When my dad would come home from work during the spring and summer, I would ask him to hit me some fly balls outside. The fact that he was tired from a long day of work wasn't that recognizable by me.

When I was able to buy my own car I wanted a sports car. Prior to this my parents had let me periodically use my dad's little orange-colored Ford Maverick Grabber special with a neat black side stripe and decorative hood. After my father passed away, my mother let me use this car. I drove it back and forth to college. Over the course of a number of years, I had four different Camaros. The last two were white and the first two were yellow. I thought nothing of getting in and out of these cars.

I played a lot of baseball and softball. I enjoyed being an outfielder and had a pretty strong throwing arm. I rarely warmed up properly. It just seemed to loosen up pretty quickly and I loved throwing out base runners during games. I played what I refer to as *melon ball* and the coach would have us regularly throw the ball to second, third, and sometimes directly to home plate. One time, I felt such a level of soreness in my arm that I hoped that the next few balls weren't hit my way. This began appearing more and more and my baseball playing days were coming to an end. The point is that I took throwing a baseball (and later, throwing a dart) for granted.

I liked cooking out on the grill on either a beautiful afternoon or a pleasant evening. Bending over the grill was no big deal. Getting down on a knee to check on something outside or in the garage was pretty much the spur of the moment. If something fell in the house, I'd simply bend down and pick it up. Heck, we all drop things from time to time too.

I'm living in my third different house since moving away from my parents' home. Prior to this, I lived in an upstairs apartment in Green Bay, another upstairs apartment in Berlin, Wisconsin, and after recovering from a car accident there, I relocated to a trailer court. Five of the six living arrangements included a number of steps to regularly climb. With the exception of the first and third places I worked at after college, the others involved regularly navigating a number of steps throughout the respective facilities. I had some issues with heel spurs for a time at my second to last place of employment. During this time, my office was located on the third floor. At my final place of employment, my office was on the second floor, but there were probably thirty steps that needed to be dealt with frequently because I got into the plant quite a bit and went to lunch every day with a couple of coworkers. I went through a period of unrecognized and therefore, uncontrolled Graves' disease (hyperthyroidism) where I consistently found myself having a very difficult time climbing those steps. I would be out of breath, with a racing heartbeat by the time I reached the top. Other than during specific times, I didn't have a big issue with climbing stairs.

I had taken watching a TV show for granted until I was diagnosed with vertical diplopia or double vision back in 2010. For that matter, I took my sight for granted until I nearly went blind in both of my eyes near the end of 2012. Taking my glasses off to both get into the shower and go to sleep at night are still significantly awakening experiences every day. You can feel like you're in a fun house of sorts. Raising my arms above shoulder height was a regular occurrence. Not only have I experienced muscle contraction but it's also gotten more and more difficult to simply do this without pain and meaningful restriction.

With the onset of this muscle disease, I've had a greater and greater difficulty getting up from seated positions. I haven't sat in any type of couch for probably five years. I've found myself compensating the best that I could. No more sitting on benches or chairs without sturdy arms (and none with casters on uncarpeted flooring). I've found it best if the chair's seat height was at least higher than the height of my knees. Then I had a fighter's chance.

Because of necessity, we purchased a dependable hydraulic lift chair in April of 2012. This became where I most commonly sat as well as regularly slept. Then in March of 2013, we thankfully found and subsequently purchased a sturdy, cushioned, counter-height chair which I use when I'm in our sun room. It safely swivels and features a wonderful circular leg rest.

I haven't been able to eat at a normal-height dining room table for quite some time now. I no longer even attempt to do so, because I likely wouldn't be able to get up. For a few years, Julie has been setting up TV tables in front of my lift chair and the nearby recliner she normally sits in when we eat at home. Close friends invited us over for an awesome meal and went out of their way to borrow a stool from their neighbor so that I would be able to both sit at their dining table and visit in their living room. We'll never forget this. I've been carrying a portable, director's-height chair in the back of my SUV since January of 2014. When we visit Julie's parents, I now need to eat at their kitchen counter. I always bring in the director's chair because it can be easily moved around for visiting too. I've brought this chair into Dairy Queen, other people's homes, and to professional baseball games. In the latter case, we purchase Americans with Disabilities Act (ADA) seats and supplant the existing folding chair with my director's chair.

We commonly hear this question when we first walk into a nice restaurant: "Would you prefer a booth or a table?" Our answer is always, "we actually need to sit at either a counter or bar-height table with accompanying higher chairs or else may we possibly eat at your bar (assuming they have one)."

With just the two of us, we like to dine out a fair amount of the time. We used to love to sit in a quaint booth or well-placed table on special occasions. For some time, we haven't been able to even consider a booth. In order to get up, my legs have to be spread about shoulder width apart. The last time we sat in a booth, I did not think I was going to be able to get up... even with assistance. I can sit at some tables, but it's honestly gotten too difficult to attempt. It may sound crazy, but there's a certain combination of seat height, table height, arm types on the chairs, and sturdiness of both chairs and table that I still can rise from, but this is steadily changing as the quadriceps and forearm muscles are wasting away. Also the flexor muscles in my hands are weakening, and my wrists are hurting more and more when I attempt to put pressure on them.

There's no kneeling down or attempting to get on the floor any more either. Steps are avoided and ramps are consistently looked for. Railings have become a basic requirement for my mobility. Bending over is limited. If I do, there needs to be something nearby to hold on to. Dressing and undressing is a process rather than a procedure. Carefully chewing my food (and having readily available liquid to drink) is a norm rather than an afterthought.

> We've learned that many of our most fundamental types of expectation have necessarily changed. Who would have thought this? Most people don't and won't until they have personal reason(s) to change.
>
> —Gary Beyer

6

"She Has the Power to Go Where No One Else Can Find Me"

I'VE ALWAYS BEEN a relatively easy-to-get-to-know person. Being an extrovert, I've probably initiated more conversations than I've avoided. I am someone who likes interacting with people and pretty much always have. I prefer being *open* rather than *closed*, but this is only when I feel comfortable with the person I'm communicating with. I've never been one to have a lot of secrets and I am usually readily approachable by others. However, I don't let a lot of people get that close to me. I would be classified as being open by nature, but my degree of openness varies with the level of trust I've established with the person(s) I'm interacting with.

We all have our introspective times. During these times, we are commonly alone and find ourselves contemplating many different things. These include reexamining specific experiences in our lives, possibly addressing some uncomfortable matters, and spending some time navigating among our innermost feelings. From time to time, there are internal spots or places we may find ourselves in which are independent of our actual spatial locations. Likely, no one can truly reach us when we're there. I've often found that my wife Julie can. I believe this an extra special, symbiotic-like trait that can develop between two people whose relationship has moved beyond a certain level. There's an appreciable "feeling of oneness" for that short period of time.

I love the word "communication". I remember from my high school speech class, effective communication is only when the message intended by the sender is accurately interpreted by the desired receiver(s). Do you see how many things can go wrong here? Yet...most of us take our communication efforts for granted. Is there anything more important that we do in our lives than effectively communicating with those around us?

We're pretty frustrated if we ask for a Coke and we get a Pepsi (or vice versa). How about if we ask for a seat on the home team's side of the infield and we end up being in the outfield? Were there any emotions involved on either side of these communication efforts? Heck no! These seemed like pretty simple requests, yet they got messed up. In both cases, assumptions were made on the part of each party; the sender as well as the receiver. It seems common today for many restaurants' wait staff to interpret Coke and Pepsi as interchangeable sodas. I've always preferred Coke, but drank my share of Pepsi over the years too. I finally found myself specifically asking if the particular restaurant served Coke. If not, I asked for an iced tea instead. I no longer choose to drink any type of cola; so this communication challenge has gone by the wayside.

What I'm also distinguishing here is the impact that learned behavior has on our communication efforts. Effective communication becomes kind of like, "where do we want to go and how do we best get there." We don't just get into our vehicle and drive. Rather, before we attempt to get inside we devise a game plan in advance (albeit a very simple one in many cases).

Now, let's consider another, frequently taken-for-granted aspect of human communication. It involves the (intended or unintended) incorporation of our emotions. The greater the number of people associated with a specific communication effort, the greater the challenge there is for achieving effectiveness. The less complex the message, the better our chances are.

Other things like body language, voice inflection, degree of eye contact, personalization of message, type of message, and controllable and uncontrollable extraneous factors commonly come into play. My point is that the more you both appreciate and account for the complexities involved with your communication efforts, the more likely it is that you will be pleased with the results.

We find as we get older that there are a smaller and smaller number of people that we regularly interact with. Sure, there are still many times when we find ourselves in larger groups of people, but it's always extremely important to most effectively communicate with the people who remain closest in our lives. The daily pace of most people's lives has been steadily increasing for quite some time. It's reached a point where a number of long-time, regular communication challenges are being approached in different manners. This is further evolving with the inclusion of more and more technology. When we feel that we're regularly communicating effectively with those around us, we need to be consciously thankful. If an advanced level of communication has developed between you and someone else, you are even more blessed.

Julie and I have fortunately communicated well with each other for a very long time. There are no hidden agendas or games being played. We often find ourselves finishing each other's sentences. However, I've also come to realize that, at times, we are able to achieve an even higher level of communication…a more subliminal and nonverbal one, if you will. I've found that Julie truly has "the power to go where no one else can find me." I strongly identify with the lyrics in the James Taylor song "Something in the Way She Moves"[10] that are identified below. I find myself becoming very emotional when I listen to it. It always really hits home with me, and the tears are ones of sincere appreciation, humility and admiration.

> There's something in the way she moves, or looks my way or calls my name, that seems to leave this troubled world behind.
> And if I'm feelin' down and blue, or troubled by some foolish game, she always seems to make me change my mind.
> And I feel fine any time she's around me now, she's around me now almost all the time.
> And if I'm well you can tell she's been with me now, she's been with me now, quite a long, long time, and I feel fine.
> Every now and then the things I lean on lose their meaning, and I find myself careening, into places that I should not let me go.
> *She has the power to go where no one else can find me*, yes and to silently remind me, of the happiness and good times that I know.
> But I said I've just got to know that…It isn't what she's got to say, or how she thinks or where she's been.
> To me the words are nice the way they sound.

---

10 From the song "Something in the Way She Moves" written by James Taylor and released on his debut album *James Taylor* in 1968.

I like to hear them best that way, it doesn't much matter what they mean.

Well, she says them mostly just to calm me down.

And I feel fine any time she's around me now, she's around me now, almost all the time.

And if I'm well you can tell that she's been with me now, she's been with me now, quite a long, long time.

Yes and I feel fine.

The term "soul mate" is commonly used. I believe its legitimacy between two people is much more uncommon, however.

—Gary Beyer

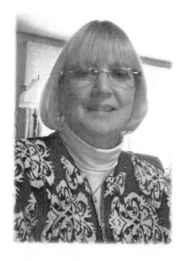

My beloved wife and caregiver, Julie

7

There Is No Known Treatment or Cure For Your Condition

Most of us have kept ourselves pretty busy over the years. We have a tendency to get quite preoccupied with many different things too. This is because our focus can be swayed from time to time by conflicting internal and external demands on our time. We don't think about something dramatically "upsetting the applecart" of our lives. We normally just keep plugging along, don't we?

Many of us find that certain life-changing events take place or circumstances arise that we are not be prepared to deal with. I often use the saying "out of the sky came a plane"[11] to describe how I felt after receiving the telephone call that January afternoon in 2008 which first confirmed my muscle-related diagnosis. I was emotionally blown away for about an hour and a half afterward.

———

Problem-solving? I used to be pretty good at it when I worked as an accountant in the corporate world. Debits always have to equal credits, but sometimes it's important to think outside of the box too. My background is in operations accounting. I've learned to appreciate the existence of different shades of gray in problem-solving because there were a number of circumstances where narrowing things to black or white was definitely inappropriate.

Resolving many of the things we encounter in our lives is simply not "cut and dried" or merely "a matter of course." We try to use a logical approach, whenever possible, but the results may be less predictable. A number

———

11 "From out of the clear blue of the western sky comes Sky King" was the popular opening phrase to a television aviation series which aired from 1951 to 1962 called *Sky King*. It was both an American radio and TV series. The radio show began in 1946 and was based on a story by Roy Winsor, the brainchild of Robert Morris Burtt and Wilfred Gibbs Moore, who also created Captain Midnight. Several actors played the part of Sky, including Earl Nightingale and John Reed King. From Wikipedia, the free encyclopedia (Redirected from *Sky King*)

of things may give us reason for consternation, but we commonly figure them out.

When you're given a message which, in no uncertain terms, declares, "There is no known treatment or cure for your condition," it gives you pause. There was no gray here, rather, it was quite black and white. Would this get your attention? It sure did mine…and very quickly too. The neuromuscular specialist on the telephone proceeded to tell me that inclusion body myositis was a progressive and debilitating muscle disease. These are the types of things that happen to other people, right? Heck, I was only fifty-four at the time. Then again, what about those people who are given this type of message in their thirties, or in their teens or are challenged to move beyond it since birth?

> It can happen to you. It can happen to me
> It can happen to everyone eventually
> As you happen to say It can happen today As it happens
> It happens in every way[12]

The specialist's matter-of-fact call to me was very unsettling. This was recognized as a substantial problem that I had no ideas on how to solve, let alone attempt to solve. My wife was at work and likely in the middle of teaching a class. The first person I wanted to call was

---

12   Partial lyrics from the song "It Can Happen" by the progressive rock band Yes, from their 1983 album entitled *90125*. It was released as the third single from that album. En.wikipedia.org

my wonderful sister-in-law, Shirley. My brother Doug had passed away in September of 2006, and she was so supportive of him during some extremely difficult times. For all practical purposes, she was a sister to me, because she and Doug were married before I was born.

I did my best to gather my thoughts after contacting two other people that I have a ton of respect for. Like Shirley, they were each supportive, encouraging, and faith-centered. I expected them to be. I'd picked up our little dog Chelsea and gave her a big hug. However, it was time again to think outside the box. Within this same short time frame, I decided to call for an appointment to meet with a homeopath here in town. My brother had been to see Nicki in the not-too-distant past. He respected her input. She was booked up until June, but I thankfully took that first available slot. Traditional medicine had made their obliging call, but it was highly clinical and not at all encouraging in nature. I was reaching out to find alternatives to what felt like a death row-like sentence at the time. The thought of my muscles becoming progressively more stonelike was not a pleasant one. Only twenty minutes after I'd gotten off the call with the homeopath's office, I received a follow up call from them. They'd just gotten a cancellation for early February and asked me if I wanted to take that slot instead. By the grace of God, this cancellation took place when it did. I was so excited to be able to get in to see her in just over a month. I took this as a very positive sign.

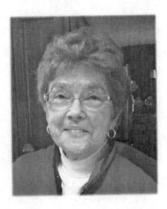

Shirley in January of 2015

When my wife got home from work (about two hours later), she was my rock. Thankfully, I have a very strong faith and I believed it was very important to get my head in the right place as soon as possible. The time frame I set for this was by Monday morning and I succeeded with this by Tuesday morning. It was time to circle the wagons, so to speak, and communicate this diagnosis to my remaining small family and my treasured friends.

Chelsea died two months later and this was very difficult because she had been "our wonderful little girl" for the past sixteen years. We met a bit later in our lives and have no children. I did my best to continue to research this disease as much as possible. It was readily apparent that nothing had been found to effectively treat it, let alone cure it. Inclusion body myositis or IBM first came into being as a disease in the eighties. Its definition was to flip-flop over the years between an autoimmune disease and a degenerative one. At this time, it is considered to be an indistinguishable combination of both.

My exposure to homeopathic medicine since my foreboding diagnosis has truly been exceptional. It continues to be a welcome breath of fresh air. I've found Nicki to be an extremely intelligent, exceedingly competent and genuinely compassionate health care practitioner. Her considerable level of guidance and encouragement has helped me tremendously. She remains a major ray of hope in our lives.

In recent years, I've also been fortunate to have also found an excellent rheumatologist. I see him about every nine months. He's been easy to communicate with and definitely wouldn't be classified as clinical. It's important to stay in touch with advances in conventional medicine, but not to be exclusively dependent upon them. For example, strategic supplementation and alternative approaches are consciously aimed at the cause rather than the symptoms of various health-related issues. They are not in the realm of traditional doctrines.

Time is a limited resource that we each are given. How we chose to use this time is up to us. Once you're given a life-altering prognosis which features unenviable outcomes, minimal encouragement, and no defined attack strategies you realize that you have a formidable set of challenges ahead of you (as well as does your caregiver). Combine this with the fact there is no identified cause, no expected resolution, and no established treatment. You can chose to feel sorry for yourself and look for sympathy from others, or you can chose to be positive and genuinely encouraged and take charge of your life.

Time becomes all the more precious. You also recognize that you need to become your own advocate and all the more engaged in your approach toward living. Most importantly, don't let life just happen to you.

"Ticking away the moments that make up a dull day Fritter and waste the hours in an offhand way.

Kicking around on a piece of ground in your home town Waiting for someone or something to show you the way."[13]

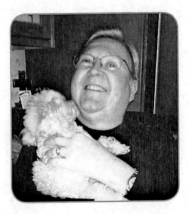

Kaylea Grace giving Gary kissies

Thankfully, I've identified a treatment which is impressively effective for this condition. It's given to me numerous times each day and night by our little angel

---

13 "Time" is the fourth track from the English progressive rock band Pink Floyd's 1973 album *The Dark Side of the Moon*, and the only song on the album credited to all four members of the band, though the lyrics were written by Roger Waters. En.wikipedia.org—Text under CC-BY-SA license.

dog, Miss Kaylea Grace. Her genuinely compassionate "kissies" are enthusiastically given and gratefully received. Are they really a treatment? I believe that they are.

> Just because you're told there's no known treatment
> or cure for your disease or condition doesn't mean
> (1) that there won't be one coming in a time
> frame where you can benefit from it or (2) that
> you can't alter your life to live effectively with it.
>
> —Gary Beyer

8

If Anyone Can Beat This, You Can

WHAT KINDS OF things bring cause for this type of comment from someone we know? We may be participating in a specific contest. There may be a race of some sort that we're about to run in. The word "beat" was consciously chosen over the word "win", however. There must not be an associated prize or award associated with this clearly encouraging comment. Whatever the cause, it is externally perceived. You are not expected to win something after completing a competition with other people. Rather, you are assigned the best chance of beating something…not someone.

What kinds of things are the reasons this type of comment is given? It's always nice to be given verbal support by our family, friends, and acquaintances. The communication of this degree of encouragement is

more than simply well-meaning consideration. As the recipient, we understand what the basis for this truly is. The associated challenge or obstacle is formidable.

When we're kids, we quickly learn the need to compete. How about for the attention and affection of our parents? This especially applies if there were other siblings growing up in our same environment. Regardless, there were times when many of us competed for the attention of a specific parent over that of our other parent. As youngsters, competing was usually associated with our attention-getting efforts.

We are commonly self-centric in our earlier years. We have a tendency to believe that the world "spins around us." Everything in the world likely has something to do with us, right? Sure, there are many other people in the world with us, but we're just basically sharing the space with them. How gracious of us.

By the time we reach middle age, most of us have "competed" for numerous different purposes in our lives. As we become older, the word "compete" takes on an entirely new level of complexity. We're no longer competing for just attention and affection. Between our twenties and forties, we regularly find ourselves competing with many different people for many different reasons. We hope to become the person selected for the job we applied for, the person who gets the promotion we believe is deserved and attainable, the person we'd like to spend our life with.

We also consistently find ourselves living amid competing demands on our time and resources. The prioritization of these demands becomes critical to our basic well-being. We strived for higher grades, but recognized that we needed to make the most of our study time because other responsibilities were regularly tugging on our time as well. What it comes down to is that we are ultimately accountable for our actions. Our behavior is not done in a vacuum. Others observe us as we go about the business of living our lives.

It's said that past performance is the best indicator of one's future performance(s). This theory is most suitably applied when a person's performance expectations are more of a controllable nature. The people that get to know us well are the most credible when making such profound statements. Shortly after I communicated to Julie (face to face) that I was formally diagnosed with inclusion body myositis, she quickly and most assertively told me, "You're going to beat this." She had just gotten home from work that Friday afternoon and, initially, she was quite shook up. As I would have expected, her tone promptly changed over to positivity and defiance. After telling close family and friends about the confirming telephone call I'd received, a handful of them made the title statement to me or something very similar to it. The cause for this level of encouragement was because they recognized that I was diagnosed with an untreatable, debilitative condition.

The reason for it was they realized that I was the type of person who was more of a fighter than a quitter and was not about to concede or give in to it.

Usually we choose our battles and confrontations. We anticipate the challenges and possible obstacles we are likely to encounter. Sometimes they come up fast and we don't have much time to adequately prepare for them. We commonly have some type of control relative to our level of involvement, but are often hampered in these efforts by our time and resource limitations. How do we react when life-changing challenges and obstacles are effectively imposed upon us? They can happen at any age and at any time. Most of these are uncontrollable. They force us to necessarily alter our behavior(s) and there's typically been no time or training to prepare us to effectively deal with them. A number of these are health related. There may be no choice but to effectively adapt while learning on the run. The most important considerations are that we face reality, figuratively get our feet on the ground and identify plans and modifications which promote success. We're not trying to win something, we're trying to beat (or effectively overcome) something.

"You cannot expect victory and plan for defeat" (Joel Osteen).

I'm determined to successfully overcome this health-related challenge. The associated obstacles are formidable, but I believe both my faith in God and the strength of my internal will enable me to be up for the ongoing challenges. I recognize that my ultimate fate is not determinable by my actions alone, but for my part, I intend to do the best that I can to beat or effectively overcome the projected outcomes associated with this nasty disease.

> The difference between the impossible and the possible, lies in a person's determination.
>
> —Former Los Angeles Dodgers Manager,
> Tommy Lasorda

9

Myositis Warriors

WE ARE GIVEN various titles and classifications in the course of our lives. Some are formal, like doctor; while others are suitably informal, like mother and father. Some are seemingly prestigious and others just simply attempt to help designate one's fulfillment of a certain role. Then there are those which dubiously surface in the course of one's handling of unexpected obstacles encountered in his/her life. Classifications like champion, survivor, and idol are indicative of achievement recognition and distinction.

This book is written with a heartfelt acknowledgement of my fellow *myositis warriors*. The classification was previously assigned with the utmost respect and it is most appropriate. We are quietly battling each day to effectively cope with a progressively humbling and functionally inhibiting condition. I've found them to be fighters in the truest sense. The associated diseases are quietly pervasive and highly impactful in the lives of both themselves and their much appreciated caregivers. The four types are known as dermatomyositis, polymyositis, juvenile myositis, and inclusion body myositis.

The terms "disabled" and "handicapped" carry with them an accompanying implication of "somewhat less able". This is not cognitively disparaging, rather, this fact is respectfully differentiated. It is because there are various limitations associated with people who are disabled or in some way handicapped. Their otherwise-unaccounted-for handicaps make them less able to do certain things that people without the identified handicaps can.

Thankfully, the environmental modifications advocated by the Americans with Disabilities Act of 1990[14] have gone a long way toward helping many less-able people become more functionally able within many environments that they otherwise wouldn't be able to participate in. We recognize that disabilities come in many different types and forms. Some are far less visible, if not even indeterminate by most people who are not around the sufferer for any length of time.

At this stage, I've found that the ramifications of inclusion body myositis are highly invisible to most people I encounter (let alone interact with). For example, they may detect something unusual in my walking gait,

---

14 "President Bush Signs ADA Changes into Law." HR.BLR. com. 2008-09-25.

but it's likely viewed as related to something other than an untreatable muscle disease. However, if they'd see me trying to get up from a normal-height chair, navigating a curb, climbing some steps (with my EZ-Step), using the bathroom (only if there's an elevated toilet or suitably located grab bar), lifting something more than about twenty pounds, or changing my clothes (especially my pants and socks), they'd wonder what was wrong. They wouldn't see me bending down to pick something up near the floor because I couldn't do it without falling. I've learned that it is of the utmost importance to be proactive and procedurally calculating in most everything I do or consider doing. Of course, Julie regularly sees the associated difficulties I'm having in completing (what most of us perceive as normal) every day tasks. The utilization of numerous adaptive devices, strategic leverage, modified facilities, alternate choices, and wise decision-making has become our necessary plan of attack.

We've had the pleasure of meeting nearly forty people in Wisconsin who are dealing with the effects of three of the four types of myositis. This includes both sufferers and their all-important caregivers. Across the United States there are currently about fifty different keep-in-touch (KIT) myositis support groups that typically meet three times per year. Julie and I have consistently found the attendees of the group we attend in Menomonee Falls, Wisconsin, to be quite upbeat and highly supportive of each other. Of the regular attendees, ten to twelve of us have been diagnosed with IBM (specifically sIBM). We are each at various stages of this progressive condition. Some are in motorized wheelchairs (with an all-important lift feature). Others of us, that remain ambulatory, utilize canes and walkers. None of the attendees are on feeding tubes, but some of us are experiencing swallowing-related issues which can eventually lead to dysphagia. It seems like most of the attendees were also formally diagnosed with sIBM in their midfifties. There are others who were diagnosed in their late sixties or early seventies. I have also established friendships with a handful of IBM sufferers living in other parts of the United States as well as one who lives in Australia. There is also an open Facebook group specifically attributable to IBM-related interests. The address is: http://www.facebook.com/groups/7950401889/

Myositis means muscle inflammation and can be caused by infection, injury, certain medicines, exercise, and chronic disease. Some of the chronic, or persistent, forms are idiopathic inflammatory myopathies. [...] "Idiopathic" means that the cause is unknown. The inflammatory myopathies are a group of diseases that involve chronic muscle inflammation, accompanied by weakness.[15]

---

15 TMA—The Myositis Association (www.myositis.org). A non-profit organization committed to helping people with inflammatory myopathies through a variety of information and support services.

Myositis is rare, affecting about ten in one million people each year. DM and PM effects mostly women in the forties and fifties, but men and children can also be affected, some at a young age (between the ages of five and fifteen).[16]

Here's a brief explanation of the four types of myositis:[17]

> *Dermatomyositis (DM)* is a connective-tissue disease related to polymyositis that is characterized by inflammation of the muscles and the skin. While DM most frequently affects the skin and muscles, it is a systemic disorder that may also affect the joints, the esophagus, the lungs, and the heart. In the United States, the incidence of DM is estimated at 5.5 cases per million people. If there are approximately 316 million people in the United States, then about 1,749 people have this disease, making it extremely rare. *Polymyositis (PM)* ("inflammation of many muscles") is a type of chronic inflammation of the muscles related to dermatomyositis and inclusion body myositis. Symptoms include pain, with marked weakness and/or loss of muscle mass in the muscles of the head, neck, torso and upper arms and legs. The hip extensors are often severely affected, leading to particular difficulty in ascending stairs and rising from a seated position. Dysphagia or other problems with esophageal motility occur

---

16 Wikipedia, the free encyclopedia
17 medical-dictionary.thefreedictionary.com/myositis

in as many as 1/3 of patients. Low grade fever and peripheral adenopathy may be present. Foot drop in one or both feet can be a symptom of advanced polymyositis and inclusion body myositis. Polymyositis is also associated with interstitial lung disease.

Juvenile myositis (JM) involves muscle weakness, skin rash, and dysphagia in children. A common characteristic of JM is the formation of calcium deposits in the muscle (calcinosis). These deposits are hard and sometimes painful lumps of calcium under the skin that appear on the child's fingers, hands, elbows, and knees. Painful sores may appear if the lumps break through the skin. The child may also suffer from contractures, which is muscle shortening that results in joints staying bent. About half of the children with JM will have pain in their muscles.

Inclusion body myositis (IBM) is an inflammatory muscle disease, characterized by slowly progressive weakness and wasting of both distal and proximal muscles, most apparent in the muscles of the arms and legs. It typically begins after age 50 and is characterized by gradual weakening of muscles throughout the body, including the wrists or fingers, development of dysphagia, and atrophy of forearms and/or thigh muscles. Unlike the other types of myositis, IBM occurs more often in men than women, and also does not respond very well to drug therapy. *There are two types: sporadic inclusion body myositis (sIBM) and hereditary inclusion body myopathy (hIBM)*. In sporadic inclusion body myositis, two processes, one autoimmune and the other degenerative, appear to occur in the muscle cells in parallel.

IBM is disabling, and most patients will require the use of an assistive device such as a cane, walker, or wheelchair. The older the patient is when contracting IBM, the more rapidly the disease progresses.[4]

Inclusion Body Myositis (IBM)

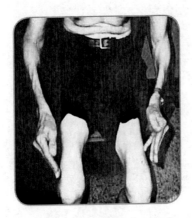

http://www.wikipedia.org/

Myositis Support & Understanding is a closed Facebook group that is intended to provide support for those with myositis or inflammatory myopathy or their direct caregivers.[18]

---

18 http://www.facebook.com/UnderstandingMyositis or Understanding Myositis.org.

National Myositis Awareness Day is September 21st.

Speaking for most other myositis warriors, we're
not looking for special sympathy. We are each
quietly doing our very best to live effectively
with our respective types of myositis and ask
only for your respect and consideration.

—Gary Beyer

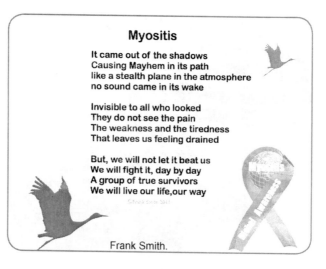

Myositis

It came out of the shadows
Causing Mayhem in its path
like a stealth plane in the atmosphere
no sound came in its wake

Invisible to all who looked
They do not see the pain
The weakness and the tiredness
That leaves us feeling drained

But, we will not let it beat us
We will fight it, day by day
A group of true survivors
We will live our life,our way

Frank Smith.

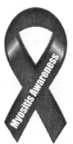

10

Stay Positive and
Be Genuinely Encouraged

WE'RE TAUGHT OVER the years to just "do the best we can" in everything we do. No one could ask for more from us. Then when failure became an issue in our lives the advice became "if at first you don't succeed, try and try again."

If the requirements for success in any efforts-based activity include the words "persistence" and "perseverance", we know the challenge is likely formidable. Such words are also associated with people who've effectively dealt with, if not overcome, difficult challenges. The latter word suggests a relatively longer time frame was involved whereby the need to overcome failure(s) along the way was probable, if not inevitable.

Facing challenges truly means addressing them. Most times, our levels of persistence and perseverance are self-defined with regard to the challenges we face. There commonly are limitations to our efforts, but it's important for each of us to recognize that the restrictions which are controllable are also self-imposed.

I've never been one to run from challenges that deserved my attention, nor did I ever pretend that difficult challenges I needed to face did not exist. Circumstances can change and challenges can become altered, but hiding from them is irresponsible. Temporary distractions can be beneficial as long as they don't become a substitute for responsibly addressing challenges that deserve our attention. Avoiding them is like refusing to admit when there are obstacles in our lives that we must get through because we cannot go around them.

What is needed in order for us to effectively deal with life's most serious challenges? Foremost, I believe the foundation for success in anything we do is an unrelenting faith in God. I've always defined true success as being happy in our lives. I believe there are two other fundamental things we need to consistently use as invaluable ammunition to help us overcome our most difficult challenges. Importantly, we can control both of them.

The first variable we can control is:

Staying positive

There are only three possible choices for each of us when we determine how we wish to approach our lives. This is a conscious choice we all make, even if some of us seemingly make it unconsciously. We can always choose to be selectively positive, negative, or apathetic in the handling of specific matters, but the overriding makeup of our personality consists of just one of the three. We need to recognize that being positive by nature is simply not good enough. We regularly encounter different challenges and obstacles which contest our positive makeup. Is it easy staying positive all the time? Heck, no. People ask me all the time, "Gary, how do you stay so positive?" I tell them, "I'm human and I don't stay positive all the time." I consciously try to most of the time, but please recognize it's okay to cry once in a while. It's okay to get upset (and sometimes angry) about something. The most important thing is that you have to return to being positive. As I regularly say, "Find your way back." Everybody's different. Such things as listening to music, reading a book or magazine, interacting with a pet, looking out the window, watching a movie, visiting with a friend, and taking a walk can help you do this. Quickly, focus on something that you find as positive in your life; something that makes you feel good. Turn your attention there for awhile.

Staying positive doesn't mean being positive 100 percent of the time. According to myself, it means being positive 95.3 percent of the time. Therefore, it's acceptable to be less than positive up to 4.7 percent of the time. We can determine the number of equivalent days this means in a normal lifetime, but you'll be a joy to be around if you can satisfy these numbers. Thankfully, this is a weighted seven-day rolling calculation that always includes our sleep time because there are times when even positive-minded people approach a less than positive weighting of 35 percent. I apologize about the geeky accounting humor...some things just stick with you and show up every once in awhile. Regardless, I hope that I've made my point.

There should be no *spin* placed on being positive and there should be no deception associated with staying positive. Concern and doubt are legitimate factors in the process of addressing challenges, but neither can be allowed to compromise our focus on positivity. I believe staying positive can be a difference maker in our lives and it's especially important when we're facing what appear to be discouraging odds.

"May your choices reflect your hopes, not your fears" (Nelson Mandela).

The second variable we can control is:

Being genuinely encouraged

All three of these words are essential to the definition of what this means. The existence of two of the traits without the other is insufficient. "Being" connotes active involvement. It reflects consciously doing or feeling something. It represents participating, rather than just sitting on the sidelines. The word "genuinely" connotes being committed. Your conviction is all-in rather than halfhearted. There is no artificiality or misrepresentation involved. Sincerity is what it's all about. Lastly "encouraged" connotes upbeat and hopeful. Failure is not presumed. Some type of success is implied. The tendency is to be steadfast in contrast to irresolute.

There is no "going through the motions" associated with this phrase. Expectations are favorable. Progress is anticipated. The wagons are being circled and we're prepared to fight on. We intend to persevere. We are not limited by our level of determination. Encouragement shouldn't be bolstered by naivety. Rather, it should be strengthened by unwavering hope. It's recognized that various obstacles and deterrents will likely be encountered along our path to effectively living with and overcoming associated challenges.

"Hope springs eternal in the human breast" (Alexander Pope).

Most importantly, we each always have these two important forms of ammunition in our arsenals. What matters is *if*, *when*, and *how* we decide to use them. Remember, they are both controllable by us and compatible with any choice we can make.

If you limit your choices only to what seems possible or reasonable, you disconnect yourself from what you truly want, and all that is left is compromise.

—Robert Fritz

11

Never Give Up

I CAN READILY attest to the fact that the advancement of this condition continues to significantly alter the way we live our lives. It is a pervasive disease which impacts so many things. I think twice (and often three times) before I attempt to do a number of things that I would, simply, have just done in the past. Does it get frustrating or discouraging? You bet it does and more times than I let on.

When you're a prideful person you never like to admit you can't do something which seems ridiculously easy to most people your age. If you drop something, you bend down and pick it up. If you need something that's on a higher shelf, you get a stepladder and take it down. When you first open up a turncap container of an orange juice, you turn it to the left, remove it, and pour the juice into a glass. Not necessarily!

Does the fact that it's become much more difficult to do many of the things that you'd always considered to be easily done make you less of a person? How about when you can no longer do some of them, if not many of them? It most certainly does not.

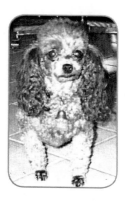

Our precious little Chelsea

When our dog Chelsea was going blind, Julie and I had a very hard time with it. She was such a dear little companion. She was "our kid" for goodness' sakes! We had her more spoiled than many people have their kids. What was especially neat about Chelsea was she was extremely well-behaved. You could let her outside without a leash and she would promptly come back in when you wanted her to. She would regularly go up and down both sets of stairs in our home with relative ease...and this was a dog with pretty short legs. She would jump to the top of our sofa to look quietly out the window for extended periods of time and also, identify *moving sunspots* on the floor where she would love to lay.

What should we do about Chelsea's condition? How could we help her or make things easier for her to safely get around? You don't put a dog down because they went blind. Yet we were very concerned for her and hated to leave her alone. At that point, we both were going to work every day. By the grace of God, Chelsea was successfully adapting to her limitations. She still seemed very happy and was clearly enjoying her life because that tail of hers would regularly wiggle and her small body found a way to avoid injury. She'd bump into things, but had both learned to slow her gait and navigate effectively around the first level of the house. Chelsea would always find her bed and there were no indications that she had given up living. Bladder cancer would eventually take her life. Medication caused some loss of fur, and she experienced some other limitations, but she never gave up.

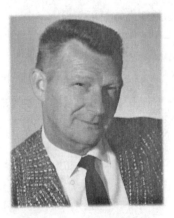

My awesome dad

When I was growing up, I saw my dad deal with colon cancer. He had a colostomy and the associated bag at his side was a constant reminder to him of his condition. I saw him writhe in pain on the living room floor from the cramps that became so ever-present with this advancing burden. He was a warrior who had a very responsible position at work. Dad also suffered from significant heart-related issues that were only controlled through medication. I distinctly remember times when it became a highly urgent matter to get a nitroglycerin tablet placed under his tongue. Open-heart surgeries were far less prevalent back then. He was never one to give up, complain, or "show you the white of his eyes." Even when he was told that he was dying, he didn't give up living. I saw this and learned a great deal from the way he handled what had to be devastating news. He was definitely looking forward to enjoying his retirement. He had hobbies and pleasant diversions. Most importantly, he didn't give up living.

My mother was a pretty healthy lady. She had periods of severe migraines, surgery for a hysterectomy, a dropped bladder, a broken arm, and cellulitis, but otherwise did not personally experience any physically major, health-related issues until she got into her mideighties. At that time, she fell by the front steps of my brother and sister-in-law's home next door and broke her right hip. Things were to spiral downward from there. Six months later, the other hip required similar surgery. She had always been a very resilient person. If anyone had true grit, my mother did. A number of people counted on her stability and wisdom over the years, including myself. Soon, she would no longer be driving, and she had been an extremely independent lady…especially after the passing of my father. They were very close and my mom stood by my dad in ways that I could never forget. She was to develop dementia which progressed into Alzheimer's. She was to live in a wonderful care facility the last four years of her life. My mother always exemplified a never-give-up mentality and she helped develop this tendency in me.

My only brother, Doug, was close to twenty-four years older than me. I'd always clarify that our difference in age was only twenty-three years and five months, but who was counting? He and my wonderful sister-in-law, Shirley, were married before I was born and ended up being married just over fifty-five years. They always did things together. Doug enjoyed life. What I'll always remember most about him is that he had a very deep appreciation for what most people would identify as the simpler things in life. He loved trees and nature. He commonly detected neat things in various environments that others would not see. I truly believe he came to learn the most important things in our lives. He dealt with numerous health-related issues in the course of his life. He nearly died of pneumonia at the age of twenty-seven, had troublesome high blood pressure, was diabetic, overcame prostate cancer, and recovered from severe, ulcerative bleeding. When he was diagnosed with cirrhosis of the liver, it became a battle that he could not win. The interactions from the considerable level of medication he was on destroyed his liver. At seventy-five, he found himself not to be a candidate for a transplant. I was at the foot of his hospital bed when a liver specialist, standing close to him, told him he was imminently dying. I'll never forget the way he responded to this statement. I'll also never forget the manner in which he regularly conducted himself after he learned that there were no options for him and that this disease was in the process of taking his life. He never gave up. He was not that type of person.

My much-loved and highly respected sister-in-law has dealt with some incredibly difficult things. Shirley has consistently proven herself to be a warrior as well. As a young child, she had a very bad bout with pneumonia, that was complicated with pleurisy, and required the insertion of a drainage tube that left an indentation and permanent scarring on her back. She's had advanced cervical cancer, colon cancer, major back surgeries, a knee replacement, and a badly broken arm... yet I've rarely heard her complain much about them. She just keeps attempting to move forward. Like my mother and my wife Julie, they steadfastly stand behind, and both emotionally and physically support, the most important person in their lives. God bless them.

When we're personally dealing with formidable health challenges, it's up to us to address these challenge(s) appropriately. We can't let others down who believe in us, and we certainly should never let ourselves down either. Feeling sorry for ourselves just doesn't get it done. "Never, never, never give up!" (Winston Churchill)

> I've often seen, firsthand, how people close to me have approached the handling of some very difficult things that surfaced in their lives. I've learned a great deal from this. There are ways to approach things and ways not to approach things. One thing is for sure…you should never give up.
>
> —Gary Beyer

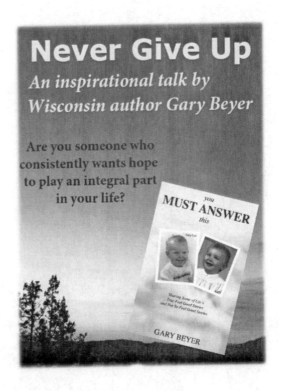

12

We'll Wait Until Spring...
Not

WHY DO WE do things when we do them? At face value, this probably seems like a pretty inane question. Many times we consciously decide they should (or need) to be done and at other times they're done rather unconscionably. Most of us are creatures of habit and like to have as much routine in our lives as possible. We try to keep our decisions simple or at least easy to determine. Also, let's wait until the time is right. We don't like things which disrupt our proverbial applecart. There can even be conflicting reasons involved in our decision-making, which further complicate matters. How about when other people are to be impacted by our decisions? Let alone possibly be hurt by them or have their life significantly altered because of them? At times, you are one of possibly multiple people that need to be involved in certain types of decisions. This can be on a personal level as well as a work-related or societal level.

There are times when extraneous variables cause us to alter our decision-making. Our best-laid plans... right? Some of these are unforeseen, but they require appropriate consideration. Others may be identified, but their perceived role in the process is initially viewed as not significant enough. Then they steadily, if not abruptly, force their way into our consciousness. Hopefully, they weren't undervalued to such a point whereby we regret a decision that was made very soon thereafter.

Some of our decisions are just more important than others. Over the years, I found myself letting the defined variables associated with these types consciously sift for awhile before making an ultimate decision. Such things as pursuing a specific education, continuing along the path of that education, pursuing a specific job opportunity, actively searching for a different job opportunity, looking for a suitable residence, changing residences, and relocating to a specific place or city. These are fundamental in nature and would be less inhibited by emotion *if* other people that you care for weren't likely also impacted.

My father died during the summer of my eighteenth birthday. I wanted to go on to college and had been considering potential options during the last few years of high school. I had initially thought about pursuing some type of schooling that would prepare me for doing play-by-play of major league baseball games or else possibly going into sports journalism. I had thought about Northwestern University in Illinois because they are known to have a strong journalism program. Thankfully for me, reality sunk in. I had basically been a homeboy growing up and was not that inclined to move very far away. I had chosen to go to nearby UW-Oshkosh and even the thought of regularly going to that campus seemed like a major life change. With the passing of my father, I also felt a strong desire to remain near my wonderful mother for awhile and support her as much as possible.

Objectivity in decision-making is great when you can find it. The greater the complexity involved in making a decision; however, the less objectivity you're likely to find. When emotions come into play, you can really have your work cut out for you. My mother was the last person to ever want to burden her children with anything and always wanted the best for them. She was fiercely independent throughout the years after my dad passed. As I think back, this had to be extremely difficult for her at many different times. Not being one to complain, she did her best to hide any conflicts she was dealing with whether they be emotional or physical. I always tried to err on the side of maintaining her independence when future decisions needed to be made.

As my mother grew older, it became more and more apparent that my brother and I needed to make some life-altering decisions that were to affect my mother. These decisions were progressively difficult too. She had lived alone in her home for twenty-seven years after my father's death and did not want to leave. Thankfully, my brother and sister-in-law lived next door. Significant work also needed to be done on the home before it could be listed for sale. Dementia was showing itself and the first consideration was definitely her ongoing safety. She reluctantly recognized that the time had come when she could no longer drive her car. Over the next handful of years, Mom was moved to a two-bedroom apartment, to an assisted living facility, to a nursing home, and lastly to a dementia/Alzheimer's facility in Oshkosh. There were a number of complications which heavily impacted associated decision-making.

We all need to recognize when it's important to move on with our lives. I wanted to meet that special person to share my life with. I am a pretty simple person and believe the range of my interests is most compatible with a more sedentary lifestyle. Traveling around the country (or even throughout a regional area) as a play-by-play announcer would not have been the right choice for me as a career. As I came to better know myself, it became clear that working as an accountant in the business world for many years was a good choice. I had the pleasure of meeting a lot of nice people and, most importantly, felt professionally challenged for most of that time.

I've always liked interacting with people. Being more of an extrovert I was comfortable in most types of social situations. However, I also was pretty shy when it came to asking women out on a date. I could talk with them fairly easily, but it commonly ended there. My sister-in-law was responsible for my meeting of a woman that I nearly married. We hit things off right away, but after becoming engaged and setting a date to be married, things proceeded to get more and more convoluted in our relationship. Thankfully, I finally made the decision to call off this intended wedding. It's unfortunate that it took a bizarre turn of events whereby I called it off at the church rehearsal the night before it was to take place. There were over three hundred people invited to the reception and we had a Caribbean cruise scheduled for a one-week delayed honeymoon. The grace of God presented a final straw to prompt my decision on the night before Valentine's Day.

I was gun-shy after this experience and also working a good amount of hours associated with work-related considerations. How do you meet that special person? I felt far from an expert. Then one summer evening, an extraneous factor took place. I was to unwittingly meet my cousin at an outdoor music festival. He was with a nice lady who he'd meet through writing a personal ad. I was impressed and made the decision to write one of my own. This (and the fact that she answered it) is thankfully the reason Julie and I met. We've now been very happily married nearly twenty-seven years.

I was living in a nice house with excellent curb appeal before we got married. Home remodeling is decided on for many different reasons. Some of the projects are pursued strictly for aesthetic purposes while others are done to improve specific functionality or add a worthwhile feature. We had added a multilevel deck to the back of this raised ranch home. There was no dining area and the home included a number of smaller rooms. There was one, small questionably placed wall in a corner of our primary living room. Even the Christmas tree looked crunched into this area. A time came when we decided to have this non-load-bearing wall knocked out. This opened up a wonderful area between the living room and an adjoining room. Part of this decision-making process was that we also recognized that a sliding patio door could be inserted into that room's outer wall whereby it would lead directly out to the second floor of the preexisting deck.

For various reasons, we later decided to look for a different home. When we were considering the purchase of another home, we tried to be as objective as possible. There were some specific factors like compatible locations and desired features that we were looking for. We had gone through some so-called parade homes over the last few years, but the original purpose was simply to get some new ideas. Before we made the decision to put an offer on this home, we identified two distinct things that we also wanted to do if we purchased it. First, we wanted to quickly change the unfinished basement into an additional living space, and second, we wanted to add a sunroom to the home's west side. The second matter was to be pursued, but likely not before a couple of years were to go by. Our offer was accepted, and we followed through with our associated decisions.

Julie and I love dogs. We were blessed to have little Chelsea (a toy poodle) in our lives for sixteen years of our marriage. We'd consciously decided to have no children of our own. When we met, Julie was already a pseudo-mom for a number of years while being a high school teacher. We decided that being parents just wasn't for us, and we've never regretted this extremely important decision. After Chelsea passed, we knew that we'd likely want to get another dog, but the timing had to be right. We believed that we would come to know when this time was right and we certainly did. We were mutually ready on that Sunday morning when we headed to Antigo, Wisconsin, to check out three toy breed poodles Julie had seen advertised in a buyer's guide. We both thought we'd be driving back with one of them as our new pal. We were right because the dog that's become little Kaylea Grace clearly stole (make that grabbed) our hearts that day.

We've always tried to make significant decisions with an appropriate level of forethought. Since being married, we consciously share responsibility in this type of decision-making. The sifting process that I referred to earlier comes more into play. I've always said that I hoped to achieve a 100 percent success rating on such decisions. There are other decisions, however, whereby the degree of sifting needs to be kept to a minimum. In such matters, I hope to achieve at least an 85 percent success rating. Spending too much time in the making of such decisions just isn't warranted or appropriate. It's easy to identify good decisions after the fact. My biggest pet peeve is associated with what I refer to as "could've, would've, should've" people. Their rhetorical comments usually start with "if only…"

One of the more significant, but not typically major, decisions I haven't talked about is the selection of a vehicle. What type of vehicle do we want, how much do want to spend, what color do we prefer, what features must it have, and later, how long do we keep driving it before we decide to look for an alternative.

I've always liked sports cars. I've never been a truck or SUV-type person. Living in Wisconsin, I've never been a convertible-type person either. Over the years it's gotten more and more difficult for me to get in and out of sports cars. I consciously progressed from two-door cars to four-door sedans. Prior to being formally diagnosed with the muscle condition, I was having difficulty getting out from a number of different vehicles, especially when I was on the passenger side. Ceiling height emerged as another issue because I found myself becoming less and less flexible.

The future inability to drive a vehicle is commonly a very real by-product of this progressive, muscle-related condition. Like for most of us at a less-advanced age, we take driving a vehicle for granted. I was having great difficulty simply getting out from the sedan I was driving. Julie and I had previously talked about my need for finding a different vehicle that I could reasonably get in and out of, but she said, "Let's wait until spring" to do so. We chose to wait for a couple of reasons (one of which was the implications of our winter weather). By January of 2014, it had reached a point in the progression of this disease where I could no longer wait. I had clearly waited as long as possible. Without actively pursuing and finding a suitable vehicle, my driving days were basically over. I promptly went online to find an attractive option. I limited myself to a reasonably used, SUV-type vehicle because there were certainly no assurances as to how long I'd be able to drive regardless of the one we'd decide on.

One morning I became really focused and expeditious in my search. I first attempted to narrow my search by creating a short list of possible makes and model options to look into. After doing so, I clearly determined my first and second choices. By the grace of God, I was able to identify a used vehicle nearby which matched my first choice. It was the type, model, and color that I was hoping to find while also satisfying the other parameters I'd carefully defined. In the course of my search, it was the only vehicle within one hundred miles which did so. It was located at a dealership in my wife's home town and was only about twenty miles away. I do not believe in coincidences! I called to make an appointment to come and see it that same afternoon. It was visually appealing, but once I attempted to get inside and proceeded to give it a test drive...I really fell in love with it. The headroom was exceptional, the driver's view was outstanding, and its handling was excellent. The next day fell on a Saturday and my wife was off of work. We drove to the dealership, met with the salesman to do another test drive, and Julie clearly appreciated my associated level of enthusiasm. Most importantly, the comparative ease with getting in and out of this well-designed, high profile vehicle was to eliminate what had turned into a major obstacle for me in traveling anywhere. We thankfully drove back home in this functionally compatible AWD Nissan Rogue after trading in what had undeniably become a practically unusable option for me. I believe this was meant to be, even though it was not the most desirable time to be changing vehicles in Wisconsin.

We commonly depend on our best-laid plans when our decisions are less simplistic. There aren't a lot of surefire plans that support a 100 percent success rating on a decision to start one's own business prior to considering a major career change just before the age of fifty (or for that matter…at any age). I intentionally did this and am very glad that I did. However, I've come to the conclusion that we have to always be ready to modify even our best-laid plans. Unfortunately, sometimes the time frame for doing so is immediate.

Patience is a virtue, but sometimes our sense
of urgency deservedly needs to trump it.

—Gary Beyer

13

Your Caregiver's World Changes Too

I'VE NEVER WANTED to burden anyone else with any of my problems. I always viewed this as a sign of weakness. Regardless, it seemed like people were always there to help me if needed.

The parameters associated with a healthy marriage alter one's reluctance to share problems with another person. The effective merging of one life into two lives changes things in this regard. One partner assimilates the emotions of the other on a highly regular basis. After I was diagnosed with IBM, another dynamic began to emerge in our lives. The traditional husband and wife roles became burdened with a major complication. I was being transformed into a sufferer and Julie into a caregiver. I asked her to write this chapter because I believe it's very important that others recognize the ramifications my advancing health complications have been having on her life.

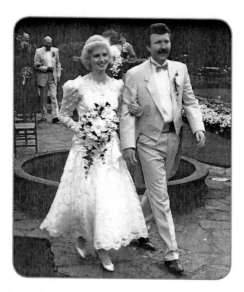

Julie and Gary just shortly after their wedding

When Gary and I were married in the Formal Garden at the Paine Art Center on October 1st, 1988, we purposefully chose the traditional Christian vows: "to love, honor, and cherish each other for the rest of our lives… in sickness and in health, till death do us part." It has now been almost twenty-eight years later and these vows resonate with me even more deeply than they did when I first spoke them. Gary has had his share of health issues over the past fourteen years or so, but the diagnosis of his inclusion body myositis in January of 2008 really threw us for a loop. Here was a disease that literally had no treatment, no cure, and was progressive and debilitating. How were we going to cope with this? How was this going to impact the rest of our lives? These were the questions that went through our heads as we drove back home to Oshkosh after meeting with Dr. Barend Lotz at UW-Health Center in Madison.

The first few years after Gary's diagnosis were not that dramatic. He was experiencing general muscle weakness and was having difficulty climbing stairs. We purchased an adjustable Sleep Number bed in June of 2008 to accommodate Gary. I also appreciated the bed because I suffer from GERD (acid reflux), and elevating my head while I sleep is a must. However, only two years later, Gary found that sleeping in a recliner was easier for him. He had difficulty getting out of bed and his sleep apnea was bothering him. Eventually in April of 2012, we purchased a lift chair for Gary. Now he didn't have to struggle to get out of a regular recliner. The lift brought him up to a standing position. This year, 2012, was a "watershed year" for Gary. In addition to purchasing the lift chair for him, we also purchased an EZ-Step (a device that cuts down the rise of a step) in May of 2013, so he could still continue to climb the stairs in our home and elsewhere. Gary's quadriceps muscles were really deteriorating and it was almost impossible for him to climb regular rise stairs. The year ended with Gary almost going blind in both of his eyes from two detached retinas. He had to have two emergency eye surgeries…one in November and the other in December.

Unfortunately, the next three years saw more muscle weakness and more adaptive devices being incorporated into Gary's life. Please refer to chapter 16 for a detailed listing and explanation of these devices and you will be overwhelmed with the number of them that are needed just for Gary to function normally. In fact, I am sure the average person has not even heard of many of them.

What really frustrates me as a spouse and caregiver is that we have footed the bill for purchasing all these devices. We were not eligible for any help from any government agency or the MDA. (Gary's condition is a type of muscular dystrophy.) By far, the most expensive and dramatic adaptive devices involved a total remodeling of our first-floor bathroom. We literally knocked out the wall between our half bath and laundry room and put in a walk-in shower, a high-rise toilet with an extra riser on the bottom (Toilevator), and appropriate grab bars. The bill for this remodel came in at almost fifteen thousand dollars! We never would have done this, if it wasn't necessary for Gary's condition.

Obviously, Gary's condition has been a drain on us financially, but it has also drained us emotionally as well. Over the years Gary developed many friends. In fact, when I first met Gary in 1987, I was amazed with the number of friends he seemed to have. We now realize that many of those "friends" are really just "acquaintances." I can count on the fingers of one hand the friends who have actually gone out of their way to regularly check on Gary either via phone or in person. With many of the rest of his "friends," it appears to be *out of sight, out of mind*. Now I realize that our modern world is extremely hectic and people have various issues they are dealing with; however, if I had a friend who I knew was diagnosed with a serious illness, I would touch base with them periodically. As a caregiver, one of my biggest frustrations is seeing my husband ignored or forgotten about. Apparently, some people are uncomfortable being around a "disabled" person. I don't understand that behavior and it really angers me. I try not to let it bother me and realize that I need to remain positive and strong for Gary. If I look at it from a philosophical perspective, I realize that Gary's condition has taught us an invaluable lesson. If you have at least one good friend in life, you are very blessed. The special friends who have regularly checked on Gary are true blessings, and I cannot thank them enough for being there for my wonderful husband in his time of need.

Being a caregiver can be a highly emotional and very isolating experience. I realize that I am literally going through the same stages of grief identified by Dr. Elizabeth Kubler Ross when someone loses a loved one to death. At the beginning of Gary's condition, I was in a numbing denial. That emotion gave way to anger/

frustration and finally to acceptance. However, I do want to stress that my acceptance of Gary's condition doesn't mean that I am throwing in the towel. I realize that certain things we were planning on doing in our retirement years are not going to happen. We dreamed of traveling to places like the British Isles or Hawaii. Gary's various health issues make this totally impractical. I want to stress that I am not mired in self-pity. Instead, I have come to a greater appreciation for the simple things we can still do together as a couple, like taking a day trip to Miller Park to watch the Milwaukee Brewers play or driving up to Green Bay to tour Lambeau Field, home of the Green Bay Packers.

Unfortunately, very few of my "friends" have reached out to check on me since I retired from teaching. Like Gary's friends, it appears that I am out of sight, out of mind. Apparently, they are either so stressed in their own lives that they don't have the time or the energy to reach out or they really are not my friends after all, just acquaintances. I always try to err on the side of positivity, so I am truly hoping the latter is not the case. That still doesn't make the social isolation go away. When someone develops a life-altering condition and is married, there are not one—but two—people who are impacted by it. Fortunately, I have met some myositis caregivers through Gary's keep-in-touch (KIT) group and they have been very supportive.

To love, honor, and cherish each other
for the rest of our lives... in sickness
and in health, till death do us part.

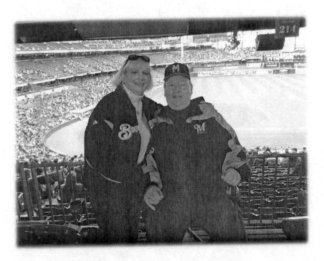

Julie and Gary before a Brewers game at
Miller Park in April of 2015.

14

Reflections of "Moonbeam" (As Told by Julie's Cousin)

WE COME ACROSS some wonderful people in the course of our lives. They cross our path in many different ways and for a number of different reasons. If we're paying attention, we can appreciably benefit from being in their company.

Some people "just stand out" as we get to know them. We find that they emanate a very appealing presence when we take the time to do so. We are truly blessed to have this opportunity, but it's up to us to recognize it. Moonbeam definitely stands out! She is one very special lady. I expressly asked her to write this chapter because I wanted it to be a part of this book. I also believed the experience of doing so would be good for her.

"Since birth, Moonbeam has been dealing admirably with a significantly imposing, life-altering condition. I've found her to be one of the most inspirational, intelligent, and well-spoken people whom I have ever met. She exudes a high degree of class and perseverance in everything she does" (Gary).

"My cousin, Moonbeam, is truly like the sister I never had. We were only two years apart in age and spent lots of time together growing up. Even today we visit with one another regularly. Moonbeam lives in a care facility in the same city where Gary and I reside" (Julie).

I was born somewhere in Wisconsin in the late 1950s. I was born prematurely, arriving ten weeks early. At birth, there was lack of oxygen to my brain. I also had a very low birth weight. I weighed only two and a half pounds. My legs were very close together. I couldn't separate them without experiencing pain and I needed help from others to do so. My parents were told that I likely had only three days or so to live, but I thankfully overcame that prognosis. I was baptized in the hospital chapel right away. I was then kept in an incubator for two months along with other premature babies. After this time, I was finally able to go home. Doctors told my parents to closely watch my development. They specifically mentioned such things as how I would hold my head up, hold a bottle, sit up and later, attempt to stand. My balance was very poor. They were concerned with my evolution from sitting, to crawling to walking.

I was able to talk in complete sentences by a year old. Being the firstborn, my mother spent a lot of time with me. She would regularly read to me and my brain was able to pick up where my legs had faltered. *At the age of eighteen months, I was diagnosed with cerebral palsy.* This is a brain disorder caused by an injury or abnormality during fetal development. It affects body movements and muscle coordination. It's usually diagnosed at an early age. It can range from minor muscle spasticity to major paralysis.[19] Cerebral palsy cannot be reliably confirmed before a person reaches eighteen months of age. During the next two years, my brain was tested for intelligence level.

People in the school system felt I would need to be placed into special education. The testing showed average intelligence. I badly wanted to go to a regular school and my parents wanted me to as well. This became very important to me. Thankfully, there were two men in the system, with considerable power, who advocated for me. They were the principal and the head of pupil services for the school district. I was glad to start kindergarten. It was the first time I'd been away from my immediate family for any length of time without outside help. It also was the first time that I felt like a regular kind of person. Half-day kindergarten was awesome. I learned

---

19 Written by Maximillian Wollner, *Everyday Health*, "Meet the World's First Ironman with Cerebral Palsy"—March 29, 2015.

to be sure to go to the bathroom each day before going to school. The severe pain in my legs continued.

During the summer between kindergarten and first grade, I went to see an orthopedic surgeon in another city. He told my parents that several muscle release procedures would need to be done over the next seven years or so. I needed to learn to be able to walk with the use of crutches. In conjunction with my significant balance-related problems, the adductor muscles in between my legs needed to be cut. Casts were placed all the way up both of my legs. Muscle testing was done up to my hips. A type of bar was placed between my legs to keep them properly positioned.

After this, I wore day braces (featuring special shoes with plates). There was metal up both sides of my legs which included straps. I also regularly wore night braces. These went all the way up to my thighs. There were different straps involved. One type was over my knees and another was attached by my hip. I needed to wear them all night, every night, after and between surgeries. It was very important that my muscle releases stayed free. This would hopefully enable them to grow with me; any type of atrophy would likely stunt my growth. I needed muscle-release surgery in both 1967 and 1972. In 1997, the severe pressure on my hands and arms from grabbing the handles and leaning forward necessitated that I have carpal tunnel surgery in both of my hands. The latter surgeries were successful and extremely important because I didn't have the use of my legs.

I completed first grade with the help of a tutor. I needed significant therapy during this time and was not able to attend school. I went back to school from second through fifth grades. In 1970 and 1971, district boundary lines changed. My two sisters and I had to go to a different grade school. This resulted in very different learning experiences. We were in the same room all day. There were huge poster boards on wheels that would have announcements on them every day. The designated class spaces, within typical classrooms, were called "pods." Books were carried in a plastic container (much like a bucket). They were then placed under the tables in brackets. I needed to be pushed from pod to pod each day. It reached a point where kids started making fun of me. They would say I was fat and looked weird. Somebody always had to push me around. I looked different outside, but I felt the same on the inside.

I wanted to go to different places and do fun things too. I often missed out on school trips. The buses at that time weren't accessible to wheelchairs. For that matter, most buildings weren't accessible either. The use of canes in these circumstances was difficult too. Going up stairs was also a problem. I'd regularly go home and do my homework. I'd also watch some TV at night... particularly shows like *The Partridge Family* and *The Brady Bunch*. I'd vicariously enjoy taking trips with them. To help get homework done I'd spend a good deal of time in the school library. Effectively, I created "my own little bubble" to live in. There was no time for any after-school activities. I had two sisters and two very busy parents.

Peers kept taunting me to the point where I didn't want to go to school anymore. I experienced bullying before this term was even created. I had nobody to play with outside for recess and nobody would sit by me at lunchtime. Through no fault of my own, I was being portrayed as a disruptive malcontent. School administration required me to see a social worker and the district's psychologist. He asked my name, about my family, about school, and if I was having troubles in school. He asked me why I was there to see him and what kind of things I did with friends. I was unresponsive to all his questions. He proceeded to ask me what kind of dreams I had and if any of them were sexual in nature. He asked if I ever think about "making it with a boy" and if I was still a virgin. I was only twelve years old at the time. Three hours later, he asked me if I had anything else to say. I disgustingly said, "Go to hell, you a-hole!" Subsequently, he put in my file that I suffered from Down syndrome.

Junior high was okay, but I had trouble keeping up with my classes. Thankfully, I had trained myself to go to the bathroom just one time per day by the time I went back to second grade. It was very inconvenient to go to the one in the nurse's office. My dad installed a vertical bar next to the toilets in each of the schools I attended. Without this, I wouldn't have been able to utilize any of the traditional school stalls. I simply couldn't fit in them.

I would hold on to this bar and pull my pants up one side at a time because of my lack of balance. Everything in this regard needed to be done one-handed.

In high school, all the main classes were on the first floor. There was an old freight elevator that went only to the second floor. It was only accessible to kids in special education classes. All the science classes were located on the third floor. This level was only accessible via stairs. To graduate from high school, I needed to get my biology credits in. As a senior, the powers that be decided to have me carried up and down these steps to attend class. Four boys were involved in this effort. Two were on each of my sides for a total of four days. There were a couple of times where we almost fell backward. There were almost 2,100 students in this school at the time. Later, a boy was assigned to push me to each of my classes. We were given permission to leave class five minutes early. Eventually, it was recommended that I complete a biology-related correspondence course to satisfy this graduation requirement. I did well with this. I could easily copy the answers from the book, but I failed the first two tests. There were nine different teachers in the science department. I was given a list of 109 biology terms to memorize. On the exam, I missed getting a B grade by two points. I was able to graduate on time with my class.

I went on to college and first tried going to one which required relocation (University of Wisconsin-Whitewater). It didn't work out very well. The

Department of Vocational Rehabilitation (DVR) encouraged me to attend a local college. The Affirmative Action Program was behind this recommendation. There were three distinct career-related options available at this college. They were: nursing, teaching, and social work. I started in May of 1978 and by 1979 I was taking the basic courses. Thankfully, this is when an Amigo (a wonderful electric scooter) came into my life. It became much easier than walking when going from class to class. By my junior and senior years, I needed to go to different locations to pursue field placements. My first one was at a place called Advocap. It is here where people with low incomes could get help with repairs, finding a job, etc. I learned a lot about resource availability there. The other placements did not go as well.

It was very hard to make friends through school. Once, I was very excited about going to Great America with three other girls. It would be fun and a great opportunity for being with other people. They were going to bring my scooter. At the last minute, they decided they didn't want to bring the scooter or a wheelchair in the car.

I got accustomed to going to and coming from school each day. The last one and a half years, I stayed in the dorm that was there. I needed to learn to take care of myself and become as self-sufficient as possible. My parents regularly took me back and forth to school before I moved into the dorm. I ended up graduating in 1983 with a bachelor's degree in social work.

There was an obvious problem which came to my attention. There was not an affordable transportation system in the city. It became clear to me that something needed to change in this regard. Thankfully, I was able to sit down with the second in command at Advocap regarding transportation issues and our conversation was recorded. That fall, I wanted to get together a group of people in the area who had disabilities. Advocap helped bring this together. There were two major issues: transportation and accessibility. In January of 1984, a group known as the Disabled Advocates was established. The one-way city transportation charge was changing from $2.50 to $4.00. This was not reasonable when many people needed to take multiple trips each week.

I found out that there was money earmarked in the transportation budget to help people with disabilities, but that this money was being used for other purposes. The Advocates group asked me to speak before the city council regarding this issue. In 1985, I was able to do that and pleaded with the members to keep the cost of intercity transportation down. The gentleman I'd talked with at Advocap was an advocate for this much-needed cost control. Another Disabled Advocates member also spoke to the council about relative statistics and equivalent successes in other places having such controls. Handi-Van service started on March 1st of 1985. We paid $.50 for a one-way ride to anywhere in the city. I was especially pleased with this because this date would have also been my father's fiftieth birthday. My dad was a major advocate for my well-being when he was alive.

I proudly served on the Housing Authority Board in my past. Others with disabilities, like myself, were experiencing some troublesome issues in our dwellings. There was an issue in some doorways. The thresholds were too high for wheelchairs and scooters to get over. Some bathroom sinks had round handles on the faucets that were difficult to turn by hand. Intercoms were attached to the wall. When people buzzed, it wasn't always feasible to get up in time to answer them. Apartment doors had big hinges which were hard to open and would snap closed. The housing authority, in my hometown, told me about a special commission in Chicago which was a sounding board for such grievances within our area. I wrote a letter to this commission and had one of my sisters type it for me. As a result of this letter, door tensions were changed to no more than five pounds, sinks were changed over to blade handles, and intercoms were removed from walls and placed in more appropriate locations. Private facilities didn't think they'd have to adhere to the rules that were in place for public facilities. They found out that they were wrong.

Over the years, I would go into schools and talk to students regarding disability-related issues. I distinctly remember a time when I went out into the hall to take a break. A nice little boy came up and asked me some questions. "Why didn't God give you good legs?" I then asked him, "Do you know where babies come from?"

and he said yes. I said that I didn't stay in my Mommy's tummy long enough and that I came too soon. I told the kids about my surgeries that were intended to enable my muscles to lengthen and make them easier to grow (and cause me less pain). The little boy said, "Why don't the doctors help you?" I said, "Some problems just don't go away." He was only about six or seven. He then sat on the ground and actually tried to pull his own legs off. He wanted me to borrow his legs. He was so upset and this truly bothered me a great deal. I came up with the idea that he could help me by reaching something for me. His eyes just lit up. I wondered what type of conversation he was going to have with his parents that evening. I'd also told him his parents had done such a good job of raising him. I'm past the point in my life to get involved with any type of volunteer work anymore. I'm at peace with that. Being in a nursing home full time, I keep myself busy enough. I regularly find time to read, to listen to music and get involved with many of the activities which are here. I still try to help others whenever I can, but it's on a more one-on-one basis. I've been on a lot of committees, but not everyone is meant to be on a committee. At times, I felt a bit less human going through a lot of the protocol and politics. Also, libraries are such an important resource and they never should be overlooked.

You can do a lot of interesting and fulfilling things behind the scenes.

In closing, the only regret I have is that nothing could ever be spontaneous in my life. Everything had to be planned at least twenty-four hours in advance. I've learned to live with my disability. I've also learned it's so important to share, understand, and care for one another. It's so important to network, network, and network until you can possibly find an answer to what your problem may be.

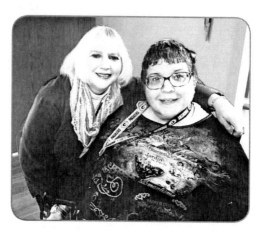

Julie and her wonderful cousin

15

Don't Let the Highs Get Too High or the Lows Get Too Low

OUR VARIOUS EMOTIONAL triggers become engaged for different reasons. For some of them, the complexity of the trigger and the reasons for their engagement change because of our age, our environments, and our life experiences. Some we believe we can control quite well, while others we recognize we have little control over.

The range of our emotions is considerable. We can realize those of extreme elation and severe depression. Some are fleeting and others seem to be lasting forever. There are catalysts which elicit an unplanned or even unexpected response. Then there are those we can successfully predict the occurrence of well in advance.

As young children, we laugh quickly at numerous different things. My brother used to spin a hat around my head when I was in a high chair and I would laugh incessantly for a few minutes. Simple body movements and facial expressions, made by others to grab our attention, would typically cause us to laugh. We'd turn sad pretty quickly too, if we felt the urge. We may have been bothered because we'd lost the attention of a parent or grandparent.

Our emotions enable us to communicate feelings without verbalizing them. They make us multidimensional within a very small space. We can sit in the same chair in front of a TV screen and watch a stand-up comedy routine, followed by a tearjerker movie, followed by a local news report. Each of these external catalysts likely caused us to realize different emotions. Commercials within these features were aimed at triggering an emotional response in us that would later cause us to react in a desired way. Of course, if one of them advertised a certain type of popcorn or pizza, we may have been inclined to simply get up from our chairs and either make a bowl or bake one for ourself.

There are times when we find ourselves living vicariously through the actions and experiences of others. It's human nature to want your children to exceed your own accomplishments. We expect them to do well in scholastics and extracurricular activities. We want our sports teams to win championships, and we want ourselves to look, dress, and act like the celebrities we admire. There is a definite degree of artificiality here because *we are not directly involved* in any of these behaviors or activities. Do these things affect our emotions? You bet they do. If our son doesn't get the grade(s) we feel he deserves or isn't in the starting lineup regularly, we can take it personally and internalize it. If our chosen baseball team isn't playing well, our moods can be significantly affected. If we believe our favorite actor is out of sorts about something, we can find ourselves being out of sorts. We allow ourselves to plunge into such diversion and be internally infiltrated because we believe living vicariously through the actions of others is one of the best ways we can achieve happiness.

We always prefer things that make us feel happy. Our degree of happiness isn't always that relevant. It sure is neat though when our happiness turns into laughter or our laughter turns into pleasure or if our pleasure turns into exhilaration. Whoa…what a neat range of emotions! Others would find that our body language and facial expressions will ride along with these developments. We like to be happy and others like to see us be happy too. We're a lot more enjoyable to be around when we're happy.

Like my mother used to say, "You have to take the bitter with the batter." No one wants to be sad about anything. Unfortunately, there will be a number of things that will make us feel sad. Rain is great for keeping the grass green and growing plants and flowers. A rainy day can trigger happiness for many reasons.

Farmers are the first to recognize that regular periods of moderate rain are necessary for them to sustain their livelihoods. However, even for them, too much rain can become devastating. In such cases, their emotional response would move well beyond sad into something much more serious.

There's a major inference in the final sentence above which is important to recognize. Our emotions don't always progress from the lowest to the highest level. There is not a protocol where we move from one phase to the next in any logical manner. Also, when we're at one of the extremes, there is no efficient way to move back to the other end of the spectrum. In the past, there were times when an alcoholic beverage would seem to help....but this was only temporary. There is no escaping our emotions and if we try to kid ourselves, we may be in for a rude awakening at a later time.

How and when we express our emotions is best reflective of "the human existence." This is what differentiates us from other living beings. You may have detected a sense of uncontrollability being inferred in many of our emotions. I believe this is only true to a point. Our experiences impact us, but (thankfully) they don't define us. As we are accountable for our actions, we are also accountable for keeping our emotions in check. There can be a tendency to "go with the flow," but doing so is not always a good thing for us to do. You've probably heard people say, "We're just going to let it run its course." Well, with emotions this is not a good decision.

Getting too high or too low on anything for very long is never a good thing. We may think it is, but we are better served if we recognize and appreciate the highs for what they are and distinguish and reconcile the lows for what they are. Extreme elation for a short period of time is a good thing. Severe depression for a short period of time is an understandable thing. We must consciously move on from both for our own well-being.

"Experience is not what happens to you; it is what you do with what happens to you" (Aldous Huxley).

The expression of our emotions takes place in conjunction with living our lives. They are vital to our existence and frequently evident in our behavior. They fuel our internal makeup and keep us interesting to others. It's desirable to normally let them flow naturally, but we must try to not let the associated highs get too high or the lows to get too low. If they happen, we must be cognizant of this fact and consciously make concerted efforts to make them more moderate. We may not be able to minimize the time frames from some of our lows, but we need to keep them in perspective as well.

> We're happy when we're happy and
> we're sad when we're sad, but we can't let
> ourselves remain enthusiastically inflated
> or stay emotionally distraught.
>
> —Gary Beyer

16

The Toilevator Grande and Other "Inanimate Friends"

I'VE BEEN REGULARLY sleeping in a hydraulic lift chair since April of 2012. A few years prior to that, I was most comfortable using a normal recliner. I had been diagnosed with sleep apnea and found it easier to breathe when I wasn't lying flat.

Sleeping in a bed at night is one of the things that most people take for granted. The advancement of my muscle condition made it imperative that I find a suitable alternative. The level of inflexibility associated with this disease has dramatically altered my overall mobility. If you'd see the way I now attempt to get out of a bed, you'd understand.

I've found the effects of inclusion body myositis to be increasingly pervasive. They impact my life in so many different ways. You can let them wear you down or you can attempt to overcome them. I chose to do my best to consciously attempt to overcome them for as long as possible.

I've always been someone who is more proactive than reactive. I've not been one to just sit back and wait for, otherwise controllable things, to disrupt my life. The "everything will be all right mentality" is not one that I adhere to. Julie has said that I can be "as tenacious as a terrier" when I attempt to get things done. I'm very proud of that personality trait.

Thankfully, thus far I've been able to identify a number of assistive devices and/or take alternative means in order to successfully accomplish most of my day-to-day activities and functions. Hopefully, a number of the things I'll be identifying below will help others as well. They've become my highly-valued "inanimate helpers." I'll affectionately call them "my thirty-somethings."

1. EZ-Step unit (this portable, extremely lightweight device features a cane attached to a stable, four-inch lift block)—This has been an absolute star performer. Without it, I wouldn't be able to navigate stairs or step onto a number of curbs. I now carry an extra one of these in my vehicle at all times.

2. Comfort-height toilet—A definite must! Even before my condition worsened to the point it

now is at, I was having more and more difficulty getting up from standard-height toilets. Such toilets are no longer an option for me (even when there's generic grab bar positioning).

3. Portable, Sutton Bridge aluminum director's-height chair— Another star! It's weight tested for six hundred pounds and weighs only fourteen pounds. It's easy to set up and expands with a nice footrest. It's in the back of my vehicle at all times. I take it with me inside numerous places where I expect to sit down (like at presentations), but don't expect them to have at least counter-height seating as an option. I need to bring it in with me at Dairy Queen.

4. Buckingham Easy Wipe and Comfort Wipe devices—These are very similar. I've experienced significant arm muscle contraction in conjunction with this condition. This device has truly been a godsend and I don't know what I'd do without it. I also carry a compact, foldable version in my vehicle at all times.

5. Hydropneumatic, Uplift seat assist—This highly portable, nonelectric product enables one to lean forward, which causes the seat portion to slowly incline to a position that will enable you to be able to stand up. It is intended to only be used on the seats of stable/sturdy chairs with arms. This version is weight tested for up to 350 pounds.

6. Hand-triggered, lightweight "grabber" devices—I'm constantly dropping things on the floor. This condition impacts one's flexor muscles and I no longer can rely on my grip or my capacity to hold onto things. I have a few of them at different locations in our house and one in our garage.

7. Elongated toilet seat riser (three and a half inches)—The comfort-height toilet was fine for awhile, but with the further weakening of my quadriceps muscles, I needed another significant toilet height adjustment.

8. Counter-level, cushioned swivel chair—We added this chair into our sun room area to provide me with another seating option. The only other comfortable chair option I could use (and always did use) was my hydraulic lift chair.

9. Elevated computer chair—I wouldn't be able to get up from the computer if I wasn't able to use this chair.

10. Accessory device to put around foot to enable me to lift it up.

11. Elongated shoe horn.

12. Hurry Cane stable walking cane—It has a suitably flexible, triangular-type base.

13. iPhone with carrying case—I need to take this with me in my pocket wherever I go (inside or outside the house). If I were to fall, this becomes my helpline to getting back on my feet by calling 9-1-1.

14. Step assist, portable platform—It's very lightweight, yet stable/sturdy. It enables me to effectively cut the rise of the step in half that exists from our sunroom into our kitchen. It acts as a type of constantly available EZ-Step. To its right, on the wall, is a strategically placed grab bar.

15. Grab bars—We now have them strategically placed in different spots in our home.

16. Counter-height kitchen stools—These were added to enable me to sit by the counter.

17. Corners of our kitchen counter area, various other corner spaces in our home and garage—Without being able to lean against one of these areas I no longer can get into or out of my pants or take off shoes.

18. Bistro-height patio table and chairs—We needed to change over from our existing patio set because I no longer was able to get up from the chairs.

19. Nissan Rogue with exceptional ceiling height—This is another thing I don't know what I'd being doing without. I've found it to be perfect in so many ways. I can still get in and out of it (even though getting in is becoming more and more of a challenge because of the increasing difficulty I have in raising my legs up…especially the right one).

20. Walk-in shower with curtain and strategically placed grab bars (done in conjunction with some major home remodeling that began in late

August of 2014)—we were faced with either moving from our home or doing some significant remodeling within it...and we both still enjoy our home. Moving may have seemed like a likely, or even logical, choice to some. However, after thoroughly considering the pros and cons associated with doing so, we both preferred to stay right where we are at this point. There wasn't a shower on the main level (where I probably spend 95 percent of my time). The location of the existing toilet was poor and had become less safe for me to attempt to use. Grab bars were to be strategically placed in the room. Advance considerations were made to accommodate wheelchair accessibility and safety-related issues. There had been two, smaller walled-in areas which made up our laundry room and a partial bathroom.

21. The Toilevator Grande (there's also a Toilevator version that is used with regular-sized toilets)— In conjunction with the remodeling, we made the conscious attempt to best utilize the existing space and retain the existing components. Cost was definitely a consideration for us. The comfort-height toilet was to be strategically moved. I found this wonderful innovation by searching online to find something which would, hopefully, enable us to raise the base of our comfort-height toilet where we would no longer

need to utilize the (more awkward) toilet seat riser. The Toilevator Grande is intended to be used with elongated toilets and effectively raises the toilet seat three and a half inches.

22. Modified garage-entry steps and the associated, sturdy railing—I currently have great difficulty with step rises that are over four inches. In fact, without using the EZ-Step I wouldn't be able to safely navigate them. As part of the remodeling efforts, we identified this as a necessary modification.

23. Foldeasy portable toilet-support frame with shoulder carrying case—This is a unit which is intended to be unfolded and placed around a toilet. It looks somewhat like an inverse walker. It gives one the potential of getting up from an, otherwise, unfeasible toilet set up. It requires the user to utilize the two side arms to help lift themselves up from the seated position.

24. Counter-height dining table and chairs.

25. Wear-over, polarized sunglasses in conjunction with prism-based eyeglasses—The diplopia-related issues I deal with are compensated for by the use of prisms. The significant degree of light sensitivity with my vision makes these wear-over glasses a necessity.

26. Flexible straws—This condition carries with it some swallowing-related issues. The use of straws makes it much easier for me to drink liquids.

27. Two-pound hand weights and squeeze balls.
28. Gait belt.
29. Expandable back scratcher.
30. Aquila lightweight, firm foam seat elevation pad—This is *not* a seat cushion. The properties of it are such that it's consciously designed to hold its shape and density. The sacral area is made especially comfortable, but the remaining area is comfortable as well. The version I'm using is 16 × 16 inches and four inches thick, but desired dimensions can be customized. There is also a shoulder strap, so it's very easy to take along with you.
31. Perfect Sleep Chair (hydraulic lift chair with massage feature)—This is an advanced type of lift chair which is designed to be used as a sleeper as well. It lays back further than the typical lift chair.

I sincerely hope this list gets in to the hands of a lot of doctors and other health care practitioners. I've consciously attempted to inform such people of items which are less mainstream with regard to their recognition. They sure help me and I know they can help others.

I don't expect or desire people to feel sorry
for me. I do, however, ask that they give some
consideration to the fact that I'm quietly dealing
with some significant limitations that may be less
visible, but they're still substantially imposing.

—Gary Beyer

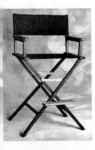

Portable SUTTON BRIDGE directors-height chair

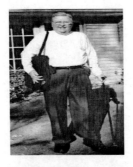

Gary w/his AQUILA Elevated Seat Pad (ESP) and Hurry-Cane

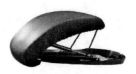

UPLIFT SEAT ASSIST
(w/hydro-pneumatic spring-assist)

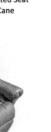

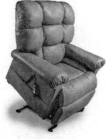

Foldeasy portable toilet support frame

The TOILEVATOR GRANDE toilet riser

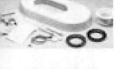

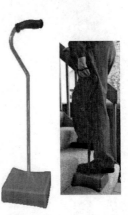

The PERFECT SLEEP CHAIR by Golden Technologies

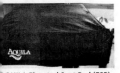

AQUILA Elevated Seat Pad (ESP)

Lightweight, adjustable & portable EZ-Step device

17

Some Close Friends' Observations

WE ALL KNOW people who are dealing with various disabilities. It's pretty special when their friends and acquaintances take the time to look beyond what their eyes can see or their perceptions can detect. These three close friends have consistently shown a high degree of interest in my well-being since I was formally diagnosed with inclusion body myositis. Their genuine compassion remains very evident and their pronounced level of consideration means more to me than my words could ever convey.

I consciously asked them to express some of their observations regarding my handling of this steadily advancing, degenerative condition. I am truly honored to recognize each of them as a close friend. With great humility, I thank them for their unwavering friendship.

When asked to contribute a snippet for inclusion in Gary's second book, I was both honored and humbled.

Gary and I came to be friends during our college days. One of Gary's high school classmates, Paul, and I became good friends in a Spanish class we had together. It is through my friendship with Paul that I was introduced to Gary. Paul, Gary, and some other friends of theirs who graduated with them from Neenah High School commuted to college daily and they affectionately became known as the "Neenah boys" as we would get together for working out, studying, and socializing when they were in town. Any get-together, sporting event, or party wouldn't have been complete without the Neenah boys.

Over the course of the years, my friendship with Gary and the rest of the Neenah boys has remained solid, as we have been good friends for over forty years. We've shared all of life's events together in each of our families including births, deaths, weddings, graduations, good times, bad times, etc.

It is with that backdrop to our friendship that Gary called me with the news that he had IBM. I, like most people, had only referenced IBM as the company that made the copier in the lounge at my workplace. Over the course of the past few years, I have been educated on this challenging and seemingly unforgiving disease.

Upon hearing the news of Gary's health condition, I investigated information on IBM along with asking Gary lots of questions about the disease and his condition.

Gary has *always* been an upbeat kind of guy. I think Gary's greatest attribute is that he's the type of individual who brings out the best in those around him because he's always positive, has a great sense of humor, is very personable, and sincerely cares about other people. He invests time and energy into making the world a better place for all those who get to know him, without placing any type of expectation or prejudice on others.

(Gary Ludwig)

I originally met Gary many years ago as a patient in my dental practice. Through our conversations at the dental office, I began to get to know him. I was impressed by his outgoing congenial nature, his depth of understanding of sports (especially baseball), his positive outlook, his determination, his sense of gratitude, and his integrity. Gary and I shared interests and most importantly, shared values.

Like many others, Gary had endured tragedy and difficulty in his life. The illnesses and passing of his parents and brother, and the challenges of the corporate world were hardships he had to face. A number of years ago, Gary's life took a different turn with the diagnosis of inclusion body myositis. More recently, he experienced the occurrence of detached retinas in both his eyes. As he went through the process of accepting and dealing with these illnesses, his life took on a new focus. Fueled by inspiration, Gary wrote a book called *You Must Answer This* and undertook speaking engagements. Through his book and numerous talks, he has helped countless people deal with difficult issues.

The concept of "there are no coincidences" and a belief in God are two things that Gary talks about often. Implied in this is the idea that we are all on a predestined mission in life determined by God. Some people are blessed with good health, family, and financial wealth. Others face daunting problems and ill health. On the face of it, one may question Gary's assertions about coincidences and God based upon the seemingly unfair lot in life that many people lead, while others have undeserved good fortune. Yet at the same time, is it possible or even likely that God has assigned us these different missions in life? Perhaps how we respond to these situations paints a larger picture of the goodness and value of humanity. Within this context, I can see both Gary's and Julie's missions in life. Their lives were predetermined to face arduous problems and together help each other and those around them.

It's not that the hardships that Gary experienced changed him into a better person, but rather in the face of those hardships he transformed his life into a life devoted to helping others. His wife, Julie, a devoted teacher for many years took on a new focus as well. Again, it's not that Gary's illnesses changed Julie, but rather through her own determination,

character, and love for Gary she transformed her
life into an equal partnership in Gary's efforts.
He could not have fulfilled his mission in life
without Julie's support, love, encouragement, and
help. Nor could Julie have fulfilled her mission
without her connection to Gary. It seems no
coincidence that these two people connected
by a shared appreciation for humanity, integrity,
compassion, and gratitude would find each other
and transform their lives.

(Dr. Gary Dubester)

We all are too quick to jump to conclusions and
label people without knowing what is going on
in their lives. Unfortunately, until something
happens to someone close to us or ourselves, we
tend to remain in our own little world.

My friend, I admire your courage, and Julie's,
and can only hope and pray for some miracle
that sees you through this ordeal. I think that
the people that take the time to read *I Promise
I'll Pay Attention* may have a new insight of what
goes on behind the scenes of people dealing with
disabilities who are not always so evident to so
many of us.

Good luck and God bless. Your friend, Bob
(Snyder)

18

Your World Becomes Smaller, But You Become More Appreciative As Well

As OUR LIVES unfold, we become more and more wide-eyed to the seemingly endless possibilities which await us. We learn to embrace the magnitude of options that we believe are there for our choosing. Through our formative years we're gearing up to take advantage of what life has to offer. How exciting this is!

We are not concerned with boundaries or limitations. That can be construed as negative thinking. We attempt to keep moving in one direction and that's forward. Sunshine, lollipops, and rainbows appear everywhere we look.

We develop one of our primary goals. This is to find a job that will pay us the kind of money that will support the lifestyle we desire. We recognize that this likely won't happen right out of the blocks, but this job must at least be a stepping stone to bigger and better things.

It can be quite the rude awakening when things don't materialize as quickly as we may have expected them to. We struggle with our patience because there weren't supposed to be any boundaries or limitations on us. Heck! We realize we can still be resilient. There's no need to minimize our expectations. We just have to find another way of meeting them. It's perceived as a big world out there, and we believe we deserve our share of it. The size of this share, however, is subject to conjecture.

It's interesting how things change over the course of our lives. We regularly experience conflicts and attempt to satisfactorily resolve them. Failures occur and we move beyond them. Many distractions are temporary and we come to expect this to be the case. Implications of disturbing matters are addressed on a case-by-case basis.

We do our best to roll with the punches and our world still feels pretty large. We may not be frequent travelers, but we get around. Numerous things are consistently part of who we are and who we've become. They're not specifically appreciated, but they're expected to be there too...without question! Our lifestyle generates these expectations.

Living large is not living beyond our means. It is living beyond our level of spiritual development. What happens when your lifestyle is forced to change and/or your habits need to be significantly altered? Sometimes this happens very quickly, if not suddenly. If you're not emotionally strong and spiritually grounded, this can be devastating. One's perception of "their world" can become significantly smaller and effectively, become more condensed.

The flow of our life has been dramatically altered since the beginning of 2008. The confirmation call telling me that I suffer from inclusion body myositis was only a formal marker for the start of the associated changes. When I think back, the noticeable level of muscle weakness I was experiencing prior to this time had already been impacting some of our decisions.

Our lives have definitely become smaller in the sense that we've consciously needed to make different choices than we'd made before this condition made its presence an issue. Its steady progression has caused us to become less mainstream, activities-wise. Some people may think we've intentionally become antisocial, but we've actually become (cognitively) antirisk. With this condition, one has to treat it with respect. It's invisible to many, but it's physically and emotionally disruptive to me. Most others who aren't dealing with some type of imposing condition do not seem to understand this. Their reality is now so much different than ours.

We recognize that our world has become smaller and that's okay. Most importantly, we've learned to appreciate things so much more. There are many things that we previously looked beyond and took for granted that we now thankfully embrace. The magnitude of options is no longer there, but that simply doesn't matter to either of us. We appreciate each other all the more and recognize that we are blessed to have gained this invaluable insight regarding life itself.

Having regular, face-to-face conversations with Kaylea Grace, watching sunsets in our backyard, enjoying nice meals at our new counter-height dining table, watching various animal activity along our wood line, listening to various types of music on our wonderful sound system at different times of the day, spending time outside, truly appreciating what our environment has to offer, embracing visits with family and friends, and being thankful for the wonderful conversations we are able to have with each other are the types of things we now appreciate more than most people could ever imagine.

The scope of our married life has become considerably smaller, but our enhanced level of appreciation for the numerous things around us has more than compensated for this fact. What a wonderful, enlightening dichotomy!

Value should not be expressed in terms of
dollars and cents. I believe it's most appreciably
expressed in line with our spiritual development.

—Gary Beyer

19

There are No Coincidences

Do YOU EVER find yourself saying, "How ironic was that?" How about, "What a coincidence that was!" You may have said, "This sure was highly unusual."

You're not alone if you did. I know that in my past I've used these phrases, or others like them, at many different times. They were the result of my experiencing some type of occurrence, situation, or circumstance which distinctly grabbed hold of my attention. The atypical nature of what had taken place seemed to be quite unusual in the larger scheme of things. There was apparent irony, but I believe it was truly predestined activity.

———

I'm of the opinion that it is far too simplistic to categorize extraordinary happenstances in our lives with the term "coincidence." This is an easy way for each of us to explain something, but it represents an injustice of sorts as well. You can stop and scratch your head, but this type of transition back to reality only minimizes our acknowledgment of what took place.

The most compelling example in my life is the interrelating circumstances which enabled me to meet Julie. I love music so I attend one of the regular Thursday evening Waterfest events which are scheduled during the summer here in Oshkosh. My cousin, Bob, was also there with a date. I believe this is the only time I ever saw Bob at Waterfest. I asked him how he met Terri, and he said she responded to a personal ad he had written in the local newspaper. This triggers me to write a personal ad (something I'd never considered doing before). I carefully write the ad and submit it. Julie reads the ad and responds to it (despite being about to conclude a difficult divorce). By the grace of God, we met. We clicked from day one and will be celebrating our twenty-eighth wedding anniversary this October 1st.

Here are some other very noteworthy examples that have been experienced during our life together:

1. My mother had lived in the home that my father and brother had built for twenty-seven years after my father's death. Over time, there were a number of issues which surfaced with regard to the maintenance of this home. Neither my brother nor myself were handy with such things. It had reached a point where we needed

some significant help to get this accomplished so that our mother could be relocated to a more appropriate residence. At that time, I was working at a business which had a more-than-capable person in charge of maintenance. We had developed a high degree of respect for each other. Long story short...he was willing and able to provide tremendous assistance in getting the necessary repair and remodeling accomplished. This enabled us to list the home and move forward with the overdue transition in my wonderful mother's life. The timing was just right to enable this to expeditiously happen. There was no coincidence here. It was the grace of God.

2. I owned a nice home before Julie and I got married. We lived there for over four and a half years after our marriage. There were various issues with it, and we considered the possibility of finding something else. We went through a number of parade homes, at different times, and tried to identify the type of place we were looking for. It was a very cold New Year's Day and we decided to take a short drive to warm up the car. We were intending to go to an annual furniture store sale in town that we'd attended in the past. Who would think we'd find our dream home in the process of taking that short drive. We had absolutely no planned intentions of heading past

the location of this home and did not even know it was there. Later that same afternoon, we were to visit it with a realtor. Recognizing significant risk, we placed an offer on this new home and it was accepted later that evening. We needed to get a short-term, bridge loan on our existing home to make this happen. We promptly placed it on the market and it was sold within a month. Were we meant to see this home on this particular cold day? We think we were.

3. I had worked exclusively in the corporate world for many years. At the ripe age of forty-nine, my last position was eliminated just a week before Christmas. I had become disgruntled with corporate-like environments, and for the first time in my life was open to another type of opportunity. The timing associated with the business opportunity I'd learned about via e-mail in March of the subsequent year couldn't have been better. Thankfully, I was open to this opportunity and had a clear head when reading it. I believe that God brought this into our lives at an incredible time. I had consciously looked into possibly buying into a small business, but had definitely not thought of looking into having our own home-based business. The timing couldn't have been better. Was this a coincidence?

4. There was the perfect timing for an opening at a wonderful dementia/Alzheimer's care facility for

my mother's needs. We'd proactively visited this place much earlier. It was a very pleasant, two-sided, small facility with about eight to ten rooms on each side. There was a significant waiting list for space availability. At the end of the year 2000, Mom's health was deteriorating very rapidly. She had quickly crossed over from living in a two-bedroom apartment, to an assisted living facility for just over a couple of months. She'd been falling, was regularly dehydrated, and was placed in the hospital only to be relocated to a different care facility. She urgently needed to be placed in a specialized dementia facility, and when I contacted the director of our chosen facility, a very nice, corner room with windows had just opened up for the first of the year.

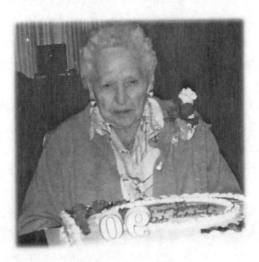

Mom's 90th birthday

Was this a coincidence? I think not. My mother had helped a lot of people over the years. Despite the trauma associated with her advancing dementia, we felt comfortable with the fact that she was able to be placed in this nice facility (which she was able to live in with dignity for just over the last four years of her life).

5. We had lost our little toy poodle, Chelsea, in March of 2008. She was sixteen and was like a child to us. People had asked us if we'd get another dog if something happened to Chelsea. We had her since she was six months old. We both knew that we likely would, but believed that God would somehow tell us when the time was right. Julie was to see an advertisement for three toy poodles in a city about one hundred miles from here. This was on a Saturday. By Sunday, we were on our way to check them out. One definitely stood out. We selected one, who was to become Kaylea Grace, ten minutes before another likely suitor of hers arrived. Miss Kaylea continues to be a huge blessing in our lives. We believe we were meant to be there at the time to bring our special little pal back home with us.

6. My mother was moved into hospice classification only about two weeks before she passed away. Her dementia had reached a stage for quite some time where our communication with her, at almost any level, seemed to be nonexistent.

Complications from a bedsore led to the timing of her death. The night before my mother's death, Julie took her hand and she looked directly at Julie and clearly said, "Take care of him." She was not using any type of sentences at that point. The next afternoon, my mother passed away and Julie was teaching at school. Was the fact that my mother made this statement to Julie when she did a coincidence? You can also judge this for yourselves. Additionally, was it a coincidence that my brother, sister-in-law, and myself were able to be by her side just prior to when she passed to tell her it was okay?

7. About six hours after plowing snow in December of 2007, I experienced some chest discomfort. As of Monday morning, it had not gone away. I was able to make an appointment to see our doctor's assistant that same afternoon. It was near the end of that appointment, when I said, "While I'm here..." It was only at this time that I brought up the weakness issues I'd been experiencing for quite some time. This lead to the determination of my muscle disease. Would I have gone to see a doctor specifically because of the weakness issues? Probably, but not for some time. Was it a coincidence that the unusual chest discomfort caused me to get to a doctor sooner than I otherwise would have?

8. During that Friday afternoon in 2008 when I received the telephone call from the specialist at the University of Wisconsin Medical Center first confirming that I had inclusion body myositis, I received, what was to become, an important call back from the homeopath's office. Only twenty minutes after I'd talked with them, they called me back to let me know of a cancellation they'd literally just received for February 11th. This date was my mother's dying day in 2005. The first chance I could get in prior to this was a date in June. She helped me a great deal over the years (and I believe she continues to). Was this a coincidence or just happenstance?

9. Was it a sure thing that I would be able to talk with my good friend and eye doctor on that Sunday morning in November of 2012 after experiencing the unusual and disturbing eye-related issue during the previous night? He urgently saw me on Monday afternoon and thoroughly checked things over. Only a couple of hours later, I was able to get in to see the eye surgeon that he'd recommended. The subsequent afternoon, I was having emergency retinal reattachment surgery in my left eye. A lot happened in a little over a day's time. I believe there was no coincidence that these things happened the way that they did. The first time I experienced this issue was during the middle of that weekend night after I woke up from sleeping.

10. When I fell in our house on a Saturday afternoon, my wife was thankfully home at the time. She was outside, but this could have happened when she wasn't around. The odds of this happening were much greater. If it happened during the week, she would have been at work. I did not have my cell phone with me at the time, and there was no way that I could have gotten up without significant help. When Julie came inside, she heard me asking for help and she quickly called 9-1-1. Was this a coincidence that this happened when she was at home? I try to keep my phone with me when I'm moving around, but when I'm in the house there are times when I inadvertently set it down some place. I hate to think about what could have happened.

I no longer believe in coincidences. There are numerous other examples I could readily provide. There have been so many things that have happened (and continue to happen) in my life that only reinforce this conviction. They aren't necessarily major things or, determinably, positive things, but I no longer miss very many of them which cross my path. I distinctly remember an intriguing conversation I had with a highly respected local realtor (named Barb) who we'd first had the good fortune of meeting in February of 2008 (shortly after I'd been diagnosed with having IBM in January) when we sat next to each other at a delayed wedding reception for our next door neighbor's daughter. She told me to "watch and you will find that God will bring the right people into your life at just the right time." I most certainly have...and find that this continues to be the case. She was right and I think of the heartfelt comment she made to me quite often. She is now a twenty-plus-years cancer survivor and has personally experienced some very difficult and emotionally trying times in the process. It's also more than interesting when you find yourself at the right place(s) and at the right time(s). If one could actually calculate the odds for some of the things which occur in our lives, we'd be stunned and in utter disbelief.

This does not infer that we should simply sit back and let things happen to us or to those we love and care for. Quite the opposite! As I've expressed earlier, *be* the featured performer in your life. Take appropriate action, be cognizant of things around you, and stay engaged both mentally and physically, however possible. I'm conscious of interacting complexities within which certain things unexpectedly come together at certain times and in certain places. There is commonly little to no predictability involved, but they are detectable by us *if we're paying attention.*

I've come to believe that there are no coincidences in our lives. It once seemed to be a sufficient explanation.

—Gary Beyer

20

What Were Once Viewed as Simple Things No Longer Are

How NEAT IS it to enjoy a freshly baked chocolate chip cookie! Okay, this goes for almost any chocolate chip cookie, but a better choice than the word "enjoy" in this question is probably the word "devour." As a child, how cool was it to have your dog treat you like you were their greatest pal in the world? You likely often reciprocated, but I bet you commonly took them for granted at various times too...until they were no longer around.

There are similarities between the term "entitlement" and the phrase "taking things for granted." Each of them carries both an assumption and an expectation along with them. A certain coldheartedness can easily be attributed to each of these words. I'm confident that you remember the parody that surrounds the word "assume."

My wife and I never had any children, but it must have been pretty cool for our parents when they watched us take our first steps. They went from dressing and feeding us, to watching us steadily outgrowing our clothes and broadening our appetites for different foods. Riding a bike was a big deal. Having a birthday party was awesome…and especially because of the associated ice cream and cake! Spending time with friends was the best.

Two of the most refreshing things we all possess as young children are our innocence and forthright behavior. Combine this with our seemingly inexhaustible energy and we usually become interesting to behold as we are growing up. As kids, we laughed when we were having fun; we played when the opportunities presented themselves and we cried when we were hurt or frustrated. Our expressions were genuine. Our manner was unencumbered and our loyalties were sincere (even though they may have appeared somewhat fleeting at times).

School came along and we became one of a group of kids. Along with this came some new dynamics. We found ourselves in our first disciplined, external environment where the primary focus was on learning and our cerebral advancement. There was one other major difference from our earliest learning environments. The related attention was no longer just on us.

As we got older, we became more and more influenced by our surroundings and the people we interacted with. Such things as music, reading, hobbies, and sports become more important parts of our lives. Our egos, frailties, and protective nature came more into play as well. We changed from doing whatever we "felt like," to doing what we thought we "should do" in the various circumstances. Choices were becoming more complex and we'd learned that undesirable ramifications may be triggered by our actions. Hey...we'd become too old to enjoy baseball cards, play with dolls, and spend too much time with our parents.

Whoa! Life had become much more complicated. Our level of nurturing had steadily decreased. Our desire to fulfill Abraham Maslow's hierarchy of needs[20] was well underway (even though we didn't realize it). We were expected to be more and more accountable for our actions and to being increasingly respectful of others around us. Goal definition brought with it some real issues and their achievement was more than difficult.

For those of us who were fortunate to meet a special partner to share our life with, I first say...congratulations! How that most special of relationships (hopefully) came about for you was likely no simple thing. It most certainly

---

20 Maslow's hierarchy of needs is a theory in psychology proposed by Abraham Maslow in his 1943 paper "A Theory of Human Motivation" in *Psychological Review Vol. 50* (4) 370–96. Retrieved from http://psychclassics.yorku.ca/Maslow/motivation.htm.

wasn't in our case. Importantly, this brought a number of (what were once seemingly) simple, but nice things along with it. How about that person regularly telling you that they loved you, or getting a well-timed kiss or hug, or sharing some intimate time with each other, or holding each other's hand while taking a short walk together or sitting next to (or near to) each other while discussing some mutually shared event or circumstance?

I've done many heartfelt presentations associated with my first book entitled *You Must Answer This*, and I consistently stress that (hopefully) we all learn that the most important and invaluable things in our lives are typically the most simple of ones. Most of these things are typically right in front of us if we don't unconsciously look beyond them. For example, going to live music concerts was typically enjoyable, but what I experienced during these times was truly so much more if I shared this experience with someone special in my life and retain the memories.

Too often we're searching for more instead of thoroughly appreciating what we have. Insatiable searches for satisfaction become unfulfilling or inadequate. Many of the most precious blessings we have in the course of our lives are unobvious at the time they appear. How about simply opening our eyes to see something or opening our mouths to talk to someone? I used to take simple things like getting up from a chair, changing clothes, climbing stairs, and using a bathroom for granted. I haven't done so for quite some time now.

The daily progression of a debilitating and humbling muscle condition has changed my life. However, I no longer look beyond most of the truly important things that I previously had unconsciously categorized as simple and commonly just took them for granted.

I appreciate all the more the precious times that I'm able to spend with Julie. Many of them are quite simplistic in nature, but they're also priceless in importance. Since she's retired, we no longer have to work around a number of extraneous obligations, albeit there are now more health-associated constraints that must be given consideration. I've come to really treasure the wonderful visits that I regularly have with close friends. They may not be defined as exciting, but they sure are extremely enjoyable and meaningful. The extensive daily "kissies" that I receive from our little dog, Kaylea Grace, are as genuinely cherished as they are fervently delivered. Going to live concerts may have become a thing of the past for us, but we still love our music. Thankfully, we're still both able to enjoy it in different ways. I no longer take reading a newspaper, watching a television, or looking out a window for granted either.

I live my life in affirmed reality, but I temper my attitude with grit. I believe that living in denial only causes greater conflict with disappointments and frustrations. I've found that living in reality brings with it some unanticipated thankfulness and genuine appreciation for numerous things I would have likely taken for granted in my past. Being a 'glass is half-full' person, a veil of gloom and disparity just can't be allowed to fit.

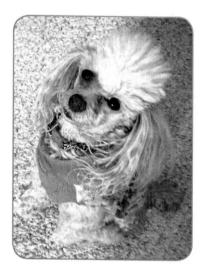

Our wonderful little Miss Kaylea Grace Beyer

One of my favorite quotes used by mother was
"Circumstances alter cases."
I also believe that wisdom and
circumstances alter our perceptions.

21

"You Are About To Go Blind In Both of Your Eyes"

"THERE ARE INDICATIONS of retinal detachments in each of them. This combination is extremely rare. Both of them will definitely require urgent surgical attention, but the most urgent involves the one in your left eye. I'm scheduled for other surgeries tomorrow at St. Vincent's Hospital in Green Bay, and you will need to be there as well."

The above was the final diagnostic step in what was to become a whirlwind couple of days. I had unexpectedly found myself, with two heavily dilated eyes, sitting directly in front of a retinal specialist/surgeon in his office that was located within the complex of my hometown hospital.

I had first started wearing glasses while I was in high school. I wouldn't have been able to pass my driver's test without them. They sure came in handy when sitting in the various lecture pits encountered during my college days. Note-taking from visual presentations sure became much easier.

I was nearsighted and right-eye dominant. I thankfully didn't need to wear the glasses for close-up work and found myself commonly taking them off and on. Over the years this would present some problems when I couldn't remember where I had placed them. I'm sure that some of you have experienced this same self-inflicted frustration.

One of my best friends, Randy, later became my eye doctor. We had sat in a couple of those lecture pits together and carpooled with another friend during our last couple of years in college. I've always had a great deal of respect for him. Julie and I have been patients of Randy's for many years. We recognize that one could never find a more thorough or competent optometrist.

Despite wearing glasses for many years, I must admit that I had taken my sight for granted. Regular testing did not detected any significant issues. I'd progressed to bifocals a number of years ago and hadn't had much difficulty with that transition. My older brother developed macular degeneration in his later years, but there were no incidences of glaucoma or other major eye-related issues in my family history. Once during Christmastime, I was trimming the tree and not wearing my glasses. I inadvertently suffered an abrasion in my right eye. As with most freak accidents, it occurred very quickly and hurt pretty bad. It was quite scary and I was fortunately able to get in to see Randy the next morning. I basically got very lucky. After this experience though, I found myself wearing my glasses most of the time.

In the summertime of 2010, I was involved in a networking group that met every two weeks. I had helped start the local version of this Northeastern Wisconsin group about two years prior. I began detecting some unusual issues with regard to my sight. Visual complexity was becoming a disturbing factor. I seemed to be experiencing some type of vertical double vision. Talk about unsettling and scary! Something highly attention-getting was happening to me and it was unavoidably impactful.

I contacted Randy and he quickly got me in for some testing. He diagnosed the condition I was experiencing as diplopia. He explained that the incorporation of prism-based lens correction would likely offset the visual complications from this issue. The challenge was to identify the correct prism configuration between the two eyes along with selecting a proper diopter size for the prisms. Randy was expeditious as usual in both pinpointing and ordering the new eyeglass prescription, but I needed to be as low-key as possible until these assistive glasses arrived. I was definitely no longer taking my sight for granted. Thankfully, the revised prescription effectively offset the diplopia issues while I was wearing the glasses. When I'd take them off, it seemed like I was in somewhat of an altered state because my vision would quickly become quite bizarre. This is disruptive to this day, but I've learned to effectively cope with any short-term implications like when showering or waking up.

I was later encouraged to visit another eye specialist to get some additional input on my eye condition. Two things came out of this visit. First, I was strongly advised to pursue cataract surgery in both my eyes. The doctor said that I had reached a point where I would definitely not be able to pass one of the fundamental vision tests used to determine the need for cataract removal. Second, he recommended that I pursue an appointment with a diplopia specialist/surgeon in Green Bay. When I met with this specialist, he made it very clear that the nature of this type of surgery was quite inexact and that it may need to be redone a few different times. This is because the eye muscles causing diplopia issues are much stronger than they actually need to be. Therefore, it's extremely difficult to determine just how much of the muscle above and/or below each of the eyes would need to be removed to most effectively improve the condition. The associated muscles had become significantly inflexible. It became clear to me that the best decision was avoid this type of surgery and be thankful for the effectiveness of the prism-based corrective lenses (while realizing that there may be a future need to alter diopter levels).

In late 2011, I clearly flunked the cataract determinant test in each eye and had associated surgery on my left eye in November and on my right eye in December. Both surgeries went very well, but a major change was to occur in conjunction with them. My visual tendencies changed from being near-sighted to becoming farsighted. Also, my eye dominance changed from my right to my left eye. I used to be able to read most things close by without wearing my glasses. This is no longer the case and has taken some time getting used to.

The previous years of bothersome eye-related issues had been very challenging to deal with. It was especially so in conjunction with the progressively deteriorating muscle-related issues I'd been dealing with. After the cataract surgeries, my eyes became even more light sensitive than they were before. It's gotten to the point, even on most overcast days, where I've found my vision to be much less stressed when I'm wearing polarized sunglasses over my regular frames. If the sun gets too bright, I now commonly close my right eye to avoid excessive squinting. When you're cognitively coping with balance-related issues anyway, the complications associated with corrective lenses containing both bifocals and prisms just add to the difficulty in satisfying normal, daily challenges. Basic, functionality type activities have definitely become increasingly more arduous.

By July of 2012, I thought that I had successfully gotten beyond my eye-related issues. Then one specific middle-of-the-night incident in early November of that year changed this. I woke up at about 3:30 a.m. and detected an unusual jagged-like figure in my left eye. I blinked a couple of times and it was still there. It didn't hurt and I went back to sleep. About an hour later, I woke up again and the figure was still there. I decided to get up from my lift chair and check things out in the bathroom. The eye wasn't red or discolored, but the flashing figure was definitely there. I then went back to sleep. Late Sunday morning, I attempted to call my friend Randy. He was very calm and definitely did not say anything to further alarm me. What he did say, however, was that he needed to see me the next day and that he'd have his receptionist give me a call in the morning to set up a time.

I drove the fifteen or so miles to my hometown to see him that next afternoon. I had the utmost confidence in his knowledge and skills. He proceeded to carefully look at both eyes and soon after dilated each of them. It seemed that he had also detected something in my right eye which didn't look right to him. He excused himself for a couple of minutes and when he came back, he asked if I'd mind driving the couple of miles to see a retinal specialist whose office was located nearby. He had called to be sure that I would be able to get in to see him that same afternoon. I said, "Sure," and headed over there. A battery of testing was completed and the surgeon came in to talk with me. After his diagnosis, I was scheduled for emergency surgery on my left eye the very next afternoon. I called my wife's school office before leaving his clinic to have them let her know. Driving back home was no fun trip because of my heavily dilated eyes. The next day was voting day. Julie had to go into work for three hours to help proctor state testing. Fortunately, she was able to come home thereafter. We went over to vote first and then she drove us to the hospital in Green Bay. The afternoon surgery went well and I was pleased to be in the recovery room. Here, I was appreciative to find not only Julie, but my good friend Gary Ludwig waiting there for me as well.

I found myself really looking forward to Thanksgiving. This first surgery was behind me and I was very grateful for the results. On the Monday before Thanksgiving, I detected an unusual soreness in the upper right side of my back. I asked Julie to check it out and she said that there was nothing she could visually detect. By Wednesday, it had become more painful and there now was additional pain in the lower front side of my torso. We went to my in-laws for Thanksgiving and I was hurting pretty bad. My father-in-law suggested that it could be shingles. It was. By Friday morning, Julie found a distinctively raised, red patch area on my back. She promptly took me to immediate care and the doctor on duty diagnosed that I definitely had shingles and prescribed some specific medicine for treatment. Thankfully, this did not surface in either of my eyes. I believe that this was likely caused because my body was on overload.

Some close time frame, follow-up visits were scheduled with the surgeon in his satellite office that was thankfully located right here in town. The left eye was coming along fine. In the meantime, I started detecting something unusual in my right eye (that was especially noticeable when I was in the shower). There wasn't a jagged-like object this time, but something clearly wasn't right. The week before Julie's Christmas break I had another follow-up appointment with the surgeon. After some regular testing on both eyes, he asked me, "Where again did we do the surgery on your left eye?" After I told him, "At St. Vincent's Hospital in Green Bay," he said, "I need to have you there again tomorrow morning." I asked him if he remembered that my wife was a teacher. I said that she'd be off the next week and could better take me then. He then said, "We can't wait until next week. You're about to go blind in your right eye. I need you to be there tomorrow."

My recovery from the right eye surgery was much longer. There were more complicated issues encountered with this one. The vision in my left eye is very good. The vision in my right eye...not so much. Thankfully, I can still see in both of them. The prism-based correction enables me to function effectively. I am very appreciative of the considerable help that I've been given to enable me to retain my sight. To my good friend, Randy, I again say thank you for your high level of professionalism, your considerable talents, and your friendship. It was because of your expeditious behavior and also that of the very capable cataract and retinal surgeons you recommended that I am successfully moving beyond these issues.

> Always be thankful for the blessings that
> you have. Everything is truly relative and
> nothing can be ever guaranteed.
>
> —Gary Beyer

22

You're Likely Influenced By Others, But Are You True To Yourself?

THE MASS MIND-SET can be pretty suggestive. Interestingly, powerful factions within that mind-set can be quite polarizing. Staying comfortably near the middle of the road, so to speak, is not always one of the available options we have to choose from.

We learn that making the most popular choice is not always the right one for us. We usually have our reasons for selecting otherwise. Regardless, it's not easy to decide on a road less traveled either. This is especially true as the perceived percentage of people selecting the most popular choice moves closer to 100 percent.

By the time we first attend school, we've had the chance to become at least one of the apples of our parents' eyes. There doesn't have to be just one apple, right? Sure, we were influenced by the other children we played with before this time, but it's at this point that we formally start the process of growing up. The concept of "having peers" was to begin generating steam. We started recognizing classmates with new tennis shoes, (slightly) older neighborhood kids with a nicer basketball than we had, and kids that maybe didn't live in as nice a neighborhood as we did.

If our friend Johnny was going to a movie on Saturday morning, we wanted to be able to go too. This didn't mean that we were actually going to go, but we believed we could go if we wanted to. Maybe we didn't even know much about the particular movie, but if he thought it was worth going to see…why wouldn't we? Since video games have become so popular, mass mind-sets frequently determine which ones are must-haves for many young adults. Identifying the latest styles in clothing is typically very easy to do because they are commonly quite trendy. You needed "to be like Mike" (which referred to wearing the same type of shoes that former basketball star Michael Jordan wears). When we're younger, the last thing most of us wanted to do was stand out among our peers. I grew up at a time when the Beatles made their presence felt in America. If you didn't have the most recent Beatles's forty-five or album, you were pretty much "out of it."

When we're young, we haven't had the time or experience to develop a financial perspective on our various desires. Heck, Mom and Dad could surely get this or that for us. If Tommy didn't keep up with the trendy clothing, it was because his parents wouldn't let him. Regardless, he wasn't viewed as cool as some of your classmates who consistently wore the latest in basketball shoes. When we come to the realization that money matters in association with many of the choices we are faced with making, we also come to that proverbial fork in the road. I'd like to choose this, but I can only choose that. There is not always a third option of choosing neither. Status quo is not always an alternative.

When we become adults, we more discernibly think through our actions, don't we? Well, at least we'd like to think that we do. This is a rite of passage. In reality, we're typically heavily influenced in our decision-making processes by others around us, and what we perceive as the best choices. These choices are commonly the most popular ones. This same tendency appears because we want to be recognized by others as being on top of things. We anticipate this same reaction from strangers as we do from friends and acquaintances. How about the dynamics associated with group behavior? Three or more people constitute a group. As humans, we are socially conscious beings. We look to become a recognizable member of, if not a respected participant in, a group. This could be a group of friends, a group of coworkers or a group of like-minded individuals. There are various reasons we choose to first, get involved and then, stay involved. It may be for our enjoyment, our self-worth, our need to belong, or because of our own insecurities. The latter keeps us in a position where we may not always be true to ourselves when associated with a specific group. When we're asked why did we do something? We respond, "We did it because everybody else in the group wanted to." How about in cases of behavioral contagion? There's not a lot of thinking going on in these types of circumstances because of the attributable copycat mentality.

Now, let's look at some intangible things. I'm consistently amazed at how many, seemingly intelligent, people become so polarized by the political party system in this country. Hatred is regularly spewed from the mouths of people on both sides of the aisle. I was always one who attempted to choose between the strengths and weaknesses of the specific people running for various positions and offices. It's gotten to the point where big money, political machines, and party pressures among peers are causing the identities of these individuals to be engulfed in the larger dogma of the party they represent. It's scary because the greater good is being determined by an extremely powerful and significantly dehumanizing methodology.

There's become a point of discussion which asks, "Who are we and what have we become?" Do we find ourselves caught up in the mainstream of activity and thought whereby we feel compelled to blend in the best that we can?

"Are we, are we Are we ourselves? Are we ourselves And do we really know?"[21]

I've always prided myself in being an independent thinker. Despite this, like most of us, I would find myself getting caught up in a larger mind-set at various times in my past. Thankfully, there were some things like the leisure suit trend that I never participated in. I was never much of a follower though. If I didn't believe in something or I didn't want to do something, regardless if my friends or most people did, I usually wouldn't do it. It's not because I was trying to be different; it's because my self-esteem was at a high enough level that I felt comfortable making contrarian choices from time to time.

Being perceived as different, controversial, or antisocial can either bring one undesired attention or cause one to effectively fall out of favor. Our consideration of such unattractive options can cause most people to simply go with the flow. Why rock the boat with your peers when it's so much easier to go along with the popular decision(s)?

Along with the steady progression of the muscle condition, I've had a lot more time to go within myself. This has only served to reinforce my independent thinking. The thought of being ostracized by your friends

---

21 These lyrics are taken from the song "Are We Ourselves?" that was written by an English rock band known as The Fixx. Their 1984 album *Phantoms* contained this song. The Fixx were formed in London in 1979.

and peers is not a good one, but empathetic friends will understand if they make the effort to probe further. I have changed in some appreciable ways, but I'm still fundamentally the same person I was before various circumstances and health-related issues necessarily altered my behavior.

> Try to realize it's all within yourself. No one else can make you change.
> And to see you're really only very small.
> And life flows on within you and without you.[22]

"To thine own self be true"[23] (William Shakespeare).

22　"Within You Without You" is a song written by George Harrison and was released on the Beatles's 1967 album, *Sgt. Pepper's Lonely Hearts Club Band.*

23　A quote from the character Polonius in William Shakespeare's *Hamlet.* (from Wikipedia)

Close Fiends, Friends and Acquaintances

I WAS ALWAYS someone whose "friends base" was pretty wide in scope. What I mean by this is that from early on my friends covered a broad array of commonly identified classifications. If I would have kept a friend's list from grade school through high school, you would find it to be highly dimensional as to the different types of kids you'd find on it.

I never liked classifying people by what was typically a very narrow categorization. We used terms like jocks, hoods, farmers, brains, studs, and geeks to identify other boys within the same school environment. Looking back, how crude and shortsighted these terms really were.

Being the child of much older parents, my mother and father wanted to be sure that I got off on the right foot socially. I was signed up for a dance class with the intentions of enhancing my development through interacting with peers and developing my coordination. I must have been more on the shy side back then, but I definitely was to become an extrovert. Getting along with people was never much of an issue for me over the years. I was never a jock or a stud or a hood. I was classified as a brain, but was close to being one of the farmers because I lived on the west side of town. There was a considerable amount of undeveloped farmland in this area. People on this side of town were comparatively viewed as the sisters and brothers of the poor. The greatest prestige resided with those who grew up and lived on the east side.

I went to Tullar my first three years of grade school. This was pleasantly located in the midst of country living. I enjoyed it and met some very good friends there. A citywide redistricting came along whereby a handful of us were relocated to a different school called Taft. This was hard, initially, because I was no longer able to associate with some of the friends I had made. Our small group of transfers became viewed as outsiders by the existing group of clan-like fourth graders. This was probably a to-be-expected scenario, but it wasn't really that hard to break apart this apparent bond.

Junior high school brought together the students from various grade schools within the town and city of Neenah. There had been just one junior high until it became time for people in my age group to attend ninth grade. A brand, spanking new school was built on the west side and it was open for business. I was able to meet some other friends, but only went there for one year. After this, it was time to consolidate all tenth- through twelfth-grade students at the high school level.

There was a pattern developing. I believed in friend retention, but all of us were being regularly separated, regrouped and, otherwise, significantly impacted by our intervening class assignments and associated workloads (including extracurricular activities like sports, band, and forensics). The old saying of "like attracts like" was coming more into play. However, our personalities had been further developing and I'd find time to associate with the people I enjoyed being with. We may have been in different classes and had conflicting schedules during the day, but there was always after school. We'd find time to shoot some hoops, play pitcher and catcher, or throw the football around.

When it was time to leave high school, friends and other classmates needed to disseminate into their own lives. Some of us went on to college and trade schools, others went into the full-time workforce and there were others who moved away. Whoa…rude awakening, huh? Thankfully, there would be summertime to ease into this major transition. Unfortunately, I was extremely preoccupied that summer. My father was seriously ill and died in the beginning of August. I had become pretty much out of touch with many of my friends for awhile. I've found that there are circumstances in our lives which heavily impact our level of "actively participating in" friendships.

College was an entirely new experience. Friends were made in classes and also by being introduced to friends of a friend. We expand our minds and expose ourselves to more adultlike experiences. We come to see ourselves in a different light. The stewardship for our development is distinctly in our own hands. Even friendship takes on a whole new meaning. I like the phrase "depth of relationship" for classifying the types of people we interact with, whether it's regularly or quite irregularly. I've found that distance apart, societal barriers, and length of time knowing each other have little to do with the depths of our relationships. "Knowing" is the key word in the previous sentence because I believe people can come to know each other very well in a much shorter length of time than we normally envision. There are some people we've interacted with for a long time and still feel like we don't know them.

There were some great friends I made after college. It was a time in our lives when we are doing our best to find our respective niches, establish ourselves in the outside world, and cognitively enjoy life. Our relationships were developed in the bars, at music events, and by attending many of the same social gatherings and activities. Meaningful bonds were created. We'd always find time to do things with each other because we enjoyed each other's company. A key focal point of these relationships was "having fun." We experienced a lot of memorable things and enjoyable times together.

We find that we have close friends, friends, and acquaintances. Importantly, "friendship" is always a two-way street, but the determination of these classifications is necessarily done by the beholder. This is because these distinctions are perception based. We find that a person's actions always speak louder than their words. This applies to ourself as well. Relationships can and do change between these three classifications. They may even be perceived differently by one side than the other. We can't make ourselves feel differently than what our experiences within a relationship tell us. Various things can cause any of us to change behaviors, attitudes, and perceptions. Some of our relationships can become positively or negatively altered by them.

I've worked at a number of different companies in the corporate world over the years. I've had the pleasure of working with many nice people. Most of those years were as a supervisor. I regularly interacted with a number of different departments and found many others with amenable personalities. There were those who periodically had divergent mind-sets too. Some became friends and others were simply "working at the same place, at the same time" acquaintances. Only a few from this past have become long-term friends.

After starting a home-based business, Julie and I had the pleasure of getting to know many others around the country who pursued the same business. We found most of them to be very nice people who were willing to assume similar risks. A number of them became friends and many others became acquaintances. A half dozen or so remain as good friends.

If we have a handful of close friends during the various periods of our lives, we are very fortunate. If we have one or more special friends we are extremely honored. If we have a friend who is our soul mate, we are tremendously blessed. However, we should be very thankful for all our friends. The treasured relationships we have with each of them are invaluable. The phrase "what can you do for me lately?" is not associated with friendship. It is associated with pseudo- friends or artificial ones. With those people, when we're out of their sight, we're out of their minds. We find that we encounter a number of pseudo-friends in the course our lives. We have an apparent, meaningful friendship, but the depth of the relationship inevitably exposes its ephemeral nature. We also appreciate our acquaintances and recognize their place in our lives. I've found many acquaintances to be highly considerate, compassionate, and genuinely well-meaning.

"Friendship is always a sweet responsibility, never an opportunity" (Khalil Gibran).

The depths of our relationships are given even greater clarity when we are dealing with very difficult matters. The clarity can really become magnified when circumstances in our lives "place us out of the loop," so to speak. We can fall out of consideration and favor through no fault of our own. Such things as health complications, financial issues, and job requirements can all cause us to make alternative decisions than we had made prior to their life-changing influence. People's concern for others becomes less dispersed when fun and lighthearted behavior becomes a predominant focus in their lives. There's only so much time and energy and it needs to be optimized, or at least more selectively applied.

"Lots of people want to ride with you in the limo, but what you want is someone who will take the bus with you when the limo breaks down" (Oprah Winfrey)

I've always liked having conversations with different people and I still do. I find this very enjoyable. It usually doesn't matter what the subject matter is. Mutual respect is always pretty special. It goes beyond acknowledging friendship. I have periodic conversations with close friends that I'm able to both see in person and only talk with on the telephone. Some are more in-depth; while others are quite light. There are times when our conversations resolve many of the world's issues and there are other times when we determine what it will take for the Milwaukee Brewers baseball team to get to the World Series again. With such friends it doesn't matter that significant time may have passed since we last visited or saw each other. We've gotten to know each other well enough that our conversations typically pick up close to where they last left off. It's neat when you detect a mutual appreciation for the time you spend together, regardless if it be in person.

There should always be appreciable room in our lives for close friends, friends, and acquaintances. We all have relationships of different depths. Not to minimize their value in any way, but we recognize the distinguishing characteristics of each. When someone becomes significantly impacted by hardship or adversity, they'll experience important distinctions between close friends, friends, and those who may have become more friend-like. Health complications have compelled us to change our behavior. It's been interesting to observe and disappointing to realize how some of the people we know have reacted since my considerable health-related issues have imposed their will over the last few years. Many of the subsequent decisions we've made (and are continually making) are attributable to addressing life-altering challenges associated with this progressive muscle disease. As pervasive as it truly is, it's been seemingly invisible to most others. The significant vision-related issues have been as well. Some take the time to inquire and show interest, while others seem to have moved on with their own busy lives.

I believe handling friendships is similar to the approach you take when teaching. Effective teachers, like my wife, Julie, attempt to meet their students where they are at. We're talking about a very important awareness here. The most diligent and compassionate of friends consciously attempt to meet their friends where they are at. They also have in common the regular incorporation of what I refer to as "an effort factor" in doing so. They regularly attempt to effectively reach out. Empathetic awareness and consideration combined with associated effort is what sets this apart. This special level of friendship behavior is not only commendable… it stands out when you're blessed to be on the recipient side of its selfless efforts.

> What would you do if I sang out of tune?
> Would you stand up and walk lout on me?
>
> —The Beatles song, *With a Little Help From My Friends* (Released on June 1, 1967)

24

Different Spins on Retirement

RETIREMENT SEEMS LIKE a pretty simple concept to understand, doesn't it? There just comes a time when our age reaches a point where we retire from working and this frees up time to do the things we'd like to do without the constraints of a job. Basically, a person consciously decides to stop doing what they've been doing over the years.

For many, the concept only becomes relevant when they approach that magical age for retirement. This has long been considered to be either sixty-two or sixty-five. It's because retirement is strictly age-based in their minds.

From Gary's perspective:

When we're young adults, retirement is the last thing most of us think about. Heck, it's such a long ways off! If it's not something that's going to impact us in the foreseeable future, it's a nonissue. Why worry about it?

For those of us who went on to college or trade school, we find out quickly that we need to learn our social security numbers. Test grade results were even posted outside of professors' offices using this number as the basis for sorting. We get into our first job and we fill out paperwork, which includes the reporting of our social security number. This is no big deal. It's common procedure, just like with the identifying of our address and telephone number. Our futures were ahead of us. From time to time, we'd hear people talking about their retirement or becoming retired. Such conversations could have been in a foreign language as far as we were concerned. It didn't concern us. Most of our parents weren't retired. This was only something that our grandparents were.

My first boss out of college was thirty-seven years old. Ron was a great guy, and I thoroughly enjoyed working for him. At the time, he seemed pretty old to me and he was a long ways from retirement. Over the years, I'd be expected to attend "retirement planning" presentations. Hey, at least this was a welcome break from work! I'd take the associated materials home and, at some point, file them away.

My father had passed away when I was eighteen years old. He'd been having health problems for a few years, and I wasn't included in any of the (likely) earlier retirement-type conversations.

Dad was planning on retiring after reaching the age of sixty-five. He really wanted to achieve fifty years in the foundry industry. I knew this was important to him because he started working in a foundry, full-time, at the age of fifteen. Who couldn't understand that? Major health issues had complicated this intention. Despite only being able to attend school through the eighth grade, he found himself promoted to the position of core room superintendent over three different plants. My father died only two and a half weeks after he retired. Now let me tell you...I definitely learned something very important from this.

Old Timer of the Month...

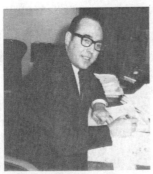

Douglas "Doug" Beyer

day wi [NE] orce of 6 men 4 wom ame the 7th n He worked with Jack Meyer and J Keating producing catalog R2. D worked as draftsman and maill then moved to the Construction S Department expediting orders loose floors and loose bench. worked several years as sales cor pondent and price estimator.

In 1962 Doug worked on the catalog, following this with resea and development duties. He assi with catalog R5. He now works in Construction Sales Engineering partment.

As a hobby, Doug plays drums v another employee in a combo ca the "Tempo-Tones." During Ch

My only brother, Doug

Later, my brother's final office position was eliminated from the company he had worked at for twenty-eight years (he started working part time there when he was fifteen). Ironically, this was the exact same company my father had worked for. My dad had worked exclusively in the plant environment. My brother was only forty-three at the time. I was getting close to turning twenty. You look at things a lot differently in your early forties than you do at twenty. However, I never forgot this, and as we both got older, I became more and more bothered by what had happened to him. I didn't work with him, but he was extremely intelligent and conscientious. He also worked long hours at various times, and I'm confident he was highly competent in what he did. Like my father, he received various promotions while functioning in different office capacities which included sales engineering and catalog management. He had gotten married young and did not go to college, but that hadn't seemed to matter.

Over the years, I regularly saw the fickle way that a number of very good people were treated in the corporate world. I worked in some form of supervisory capacity for most of those years. Long-term employees who were close to retirement, and numerous others who weren't, were unexpectedly and clinically "resigned."

I consistently internalized the different environments and personally experienced periods of satisfaction, enjoyment, fulfillment, recognition, discouragement, frustration, helplessness, and distress. After reaching the age of forty-nine, my last position was eliminated shortly before Christmas. It was done in association with a process that was initiated by the out-of-state investment bankers who owned the company. This was intended to make the company more attractive to a desired suitor.

I certainly wasn't able to retire at this point and hadn't remotely thought about it. I also had gotten pretty disillusioned with working in the corporate world. After considerable consternation and an appropriate sifting of where my head was at and with Julie's support/encouragement, I decided to pursue an attractive home-based business opportunity.

"Time for a cool change I know that it's time for a cool change Now that my life is so prearranged I know that it's time for a cool change"[24]

It was one of the best choices I ever made. It became so refreshing, stimulating, and rewarding for me. Who would have ever thought that I'd get involved with this type of thing? Neither of us had ever heard of the associated products (or the related business opportunity) until with genuine interest, and admittedly some reluctance, I responded to an intriguing e-mail I'd received. We liked the concept and found the products

---

24 Partial lyrics were taken from the song "Cool Change" by the Australian rock group Little River Band. This song was written by lead singer Glenn Shorrock. It was the second single from their sixth album, *First Under the Wire* that was released in August of 1979. en.wikipedia.org—Text under CC-BY-SA license.

Gary Beyer

to be beneficial to others (including Julie herself, who suffers from some breathing-related issues).

Around four plus years into this decision, it was becoming clear that my health-related complications were trumping what had otherwise been a sensible change of direction. Being a prideful person, I was hoping to find a worthy alternative until I could seriously consider retirement. This wasn't to be. The progressive nature of this disease and the pervasive symptoms were well in the process of making the retirement decision for me.

My retirement wasn't based on age-related factors as I'd expected it to be. It also is proceeding with many more physical restrictions and limitations than I'd imagined at any prior point in my life. I've come to internalize the old saying, "When life gives you lemons, make lemonade." I've learned to embrace my retirement (regardless of how and why it came about), appreciate the many blessings in my life, and to enjoyably live my life, amidst what's become a progressive level of restrictions and limitations.

Consistent with the text which states "objects may be closer than they appear" that is displayed on the side-view mirrors of vehicles. Our retirements may come sooner than we'd otherwise anticipate.

From Julie's perspective:

Unlike Gary, my retirement from a long career (thirty-four plus years) of being a public school teacher was my conscious decision. I had reached the common guidelines for claiming my pension benefits from the state employee trust funds. I truly enjoyed my teaching career for many years. I was a high school English teacher and also coached drama and forensics. Teaching is a very rewarding career, but also a very demanding one. Most of my weekends during the school year were spent grading papers or preparing lesson plans. The only "free time" I had was during the summer months; however, I often took continuing education graduate classes during this time.

When Gary was officially diagnosed with IBM in January of 2008, I knew that we were entering another phase of our lives. I gave some passing thought to retirement from teaching, but at that time it was not fully on my radar. However, as the years continued to pass, I noticed with growing worry that Gary was having more and more difficultly with mobility. We live in a story and a half house with all the bedrooms upstairs. I would constantly worry about Gary's safety while I was at work. In March of 2014, Gary did fall on a few short steps leading from our sunroom into the dining area. Fortunately, this happened on a Saturday and I was home at the time. Unfortunately, I was outside when it happened and came into the house to hear Gary yelling weakly, "Julie, Julie, help me, help me." With Gary's condition, once he falls, he cannot get back up without the assistance of at least two people doing a lift assist. Gary was painfully on one knee that was badly cut from his falling on the steel sliding door channel. I was able to help him move off the knee into a sitting position, but obviously could not get him upright. I decided to call 9-1-1, and a few minutes later, two paramedics arrived and brought Gary back into a standing position. They also bandaged the wound on his knee. This incident was an "aha" moment for me, and I realized that it was time to retire from teaching and focus upon being a caregiver to Gary. I composed a formal letter of retirement to submit to the school board and also started the process to begin receiving my pension fund once my employment with the school district ended. I actually planned this perfectly, and I had no lapse in payments. Once my last check from the school district ended, my monthly pension payments began to kick in. The difficult part of my retirement is health insurance. Some school districts allow retirees to remain on the district's group health insurance until Medicare begins; however, my school district did not offer that option. Gary was able to qualify for early Medicare because of his disability, but he did need to purchase a supplement. Therefore, I needed to find my own individual plan. I do have a nice plan, but I am paying more for it than I wanted. Right now, I don't want to switch, but when the annual enrollment period rolls around again, I will be looking for some less expensive options.

Although I am very thankful to be in a position to take an early retirement in chronological terms (public school teachers can retire at age fifty-seven), retirement from a full-time, very rigorous professional career after thirty-four plus years is a huge paradigm shift for me. The reality of my retirement hit me like a ton of bricks when September rolled around and another school year started. I felt like a fish out of water and had a feeling of guilt and anxiety about not being back at school. Actually, it was the first time since I was in kindergarten that I wasn't in a school environment when September rolled around. Every night for many months after that I would have what I called "school dreams." I was always back at school, in front of a classroom, teaching something like a Shakespearean drama or discussing a composition assignment with a student. I still have school dreams now and then, but not as frequently as I did during that first September of my retirement from teaching.

My retirement is not what I truly expected it to be from only a few years ago. First of all, Gary's mobility issues prevent us from traveling long distances by air, boat, bus, or train. Gary cannot get up from a regular height or lower seat. Public restrooms, even those designed for the disabled, are not functional for Gary's physical limitations. Therefore, our travel has been limited to short day trips via our Nissan Rogue. I still vividly remember an education colleague saying to me at my retirement dinner, "Enjoy your retirement, Julie! I am sure you and Gary will be spending the next cold winter on some warm, sunny beach." She obviously meant to be positive, but it created a very negative reaction with me. I didn't say anything at all. I knew the setting wasn't appropriate to make a lengthy response about why that scenario would not be a reality for my retirement.

Even though Gary and I will not be "world travelers" in our retirement, I am not overly sad or even disappointed by that reality. As Gary has mentioned in previous chapters of this book, his disability has given us the insight to appreciate the simple things in life. We have a beautiful, wooded backyard facing west. Both of us love sitting out on our bistro-height patio chairs and watching the sunset. I love feeding and watching the birds, squirrels, and other wild critters that inhabit our backyard. Also I now have more time to cook and prepare some lovely candlelit dinners for Gary and I. We recently purchased a new counter-height dining room set for just this purpose. Gary was not able to sit at our previous regular-height dining set for a number of years. We would just set up folding trays in front of my recliner and Gary's lift chair in the living room to eat in front of the television. These may seem like small, inconsequential things to the average person, but they are priceless things to Gary and I. Anything we can do to make Gary's life as normal as possible is a tremendous blessing to us.

"Retire from work, but not from life" (M. K. Soni).

> If you believe that achievement ends with
> retirement...you will slowly fade away.
> First of all, keeping the mind active is one
> way to prolong your life and to enjoy life
> to its fullest for as long as possible.
>
> —Byron Pulsifer, End Of Achievement

25

Lit'l Gar, You are Priceless to Me!

IT'S PRETTY NEAT when someone thinks enough of us to do something they believe will make us feel good. It doesn't matter how short-lived that feeling might be. This is truly a type of honor that's been consciously bestowed upon us.

As long as I've known Julie, she's always been someone who enjoys doing something she believes will make someone else happy. Her intent has always been well-meaning. I've been blessed to be at the receiving end of many of these good intentions.

I love giving friends and loved ones little surprises, "just because" gifts. Gary, my beloved husband, has been the recipient of the vast majority of these. As the effects of Gary's condition became more evident, I have increased the number of these little pick-me-ups. For instance, I purchased a chocolate bar that looked like a million-dollar note and placed it on Gary's computer desk when he was writing his first book, *You Must Answer This*. I attached a post-it note to the chocolate bar and wrote, "Lit'l Gar, you are priceless to me!" Gary was so moved when he saw this small gesture of my love that he cried tears of happiness. That's why I love Gary so deeply. He is an extremely genuine and highly sensitive person.

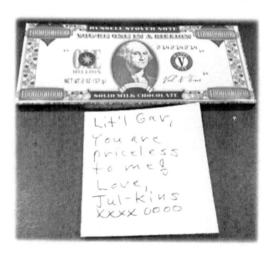

Gary and I met when I was thirty and he was thirty-four years old. We both had experienced a painful breakup of a previous, serious relationship. I actually went through a divorce and Gary called off a wedding. Both of us were looking for more than a spouse, we were looking for a soul mate to share the rest of our lives with. As Gary mentioned in his first book, *You Must Answer This*, we met in an unconventional way through writing

(Gary) and responding (Julie) to a personal ad in the local newspaper. It truly was fate or divine intervention that brought Gary and I together. I can honestly say that Gary is the perfect man for me. We have the same values/beliefs and similar likes/dislikes. Our relationship has developed to such a high level that we can literally complete each other's thoughts/sentences. Gary truly is my better half.

Needless to say, Gary's diagnosis of IBM was devastating to us at first; however, the extreme depth of our love for one another has kept us going. In fact, I can honestly say that we are truly myositis warriors. It's our undying love for one another that will be the ultimate victor against this debilitating disease. As I have said many times, "Lit'l Gar, you are priceless to me!" I am extremely proud of Gary's books and the positive message of hope against adversity they represent and illustrate.

It's not the value of the gift or surprise that's
ever matters most to me. It's the intent of
the message that is associated with it.

—Gary Beyer

26

Those Who Hope In the Lord Will Renew Their Strength (Isaiah 40:31)

GOD'S NAME CAME into our lives when most of us were very young children. We were to find out that honoring him meant more than just being in church on Sundays. We'd see various pictures of God, but learned that we wouldn't be able to visit with him on a face-to-face basis. The concept of an Almighty God was simply beyond our comprehension.

I was recently asked how important my faith was to me during a radio interview. Without any hesitation, I quickly answered, "It is huge." I also should have answered, it is omnipresent.

My parents taught me from an early age to believe in God. I was raised in the Episcopalian faith and was taught to say the Lord's Prayer every night. I would commonly get down on my knees before I went to bed and quietly pray.

We attended a beautiful church. I regularly went to Sunday school and became an acolyte. There wasn't any questioning of this reverence and respect. It was more that this seemed like the right thing to do. Looking back, I hadn't truly developed a personal relationship with God to this point.

My father developed an array of health-related issues as I was growing up, and I regularly looked to God to help him successfully overcome them. I felt very small in the big picture of life when doing so and experienced a growing degree of helplessness. I had a great deal of love and respect for my dad and it was exceedingly difficult watching him courageously deal with these very imposing matters.

Mom continued to go to church nearly every Sunday, but my father wasn't always up to it. This fact did not minimize his level of faith, however. I began to better distinguish between expressing one's faith by regularly going to church and exhibiting one's faith through various other means. I realized that God wasn't necessarily most effectively reached when in a church environment, but I thought he was best revered there. I learned that taking time to communicate with God was what it was all about. It didn't matter if you were at home, in a restaurant, or visiting grandparents.

When my father passed away, it was really hard for me. I didn't want to see him continue to suffer, but he was the type of person who loved life. I had just reached eighteen, and I wanted to spend some grown-up time with him. He had developed interests outside his demanding job. He was looking forward to his retirement and enjoying his life. He was far from extravagant and his needs were simple. He loved his wife and family. Never a complainer, he had established his own small lamp-making business and intended to pursue it further. His slogans were Beyer Lights the Dark Places and See Beyer and See Better. My dad was quick to smile and easy to get along with. The people who got to know him liked him and came to respect him a great deal.

The time of his passing just wasn't fair. He died only a couple of weeks after he retired. It wasn't fair to my mother, my brother, my sister-in-law, myself, and most importantly, him. He wasn't bothering anyone else. He was a simple soul who wanted nothing more than to enjoy his life after retirement. Fifty years in the foundry industry had taken its toll, but he was always passionate about life.

Guess what? Life isn't always fair. It wasn't a big deal if some minor things in my life weren't necessarily fair, but this was a big deal. This was the ultimate in unfairness because it was in conjunction with life and death. Another critical lesson was to be learned shortly after my father's death. That lesson is: life goes on. I came to appreciate the "just one sand pebble on the beach" concept. Specifically, that despite our identification of self, we are only one of many living in a world which is interrelational, competitive, frequently disruptive, and confusing and most importantly, it's one with shared features.

Over the years, I learned to go within myself to deal with various matters which confronted me. I'd pray to God, but in hindsight I hadn't sufficiently internalized our relationship. You see, despite being intimidated by the "just one sand pebble on the beach" concept, one needs to realize that this simply doesn't matter when it comes to our relationship with Almighty God. It may matter in worldly things, but we're talking about something which is much bigger than that. God always has time for each and every one of us. It's up to us to make the approach.

There is another important concept that I've come to fundamentally incorporate into my life. That concept is "what are you willing to do (about something)?" When we had our small, home-based business we had reached a rank where focused training and assisting others with their business development caused this to come about. During training sessions, I would consistently turn to fellow business owners and ask them this question. Simply sitting back and waiting for things to take place is usually not the best alternative. This even applies to things we believe we have little control over. At the very least, we need to stay engaged. Like my father, I've always believed that I would never expect something from others that I wouldn't expect from myself. Many of our limitations are self-imposed and it's important that we recognize this fact.

After being diagnosed with inclusion body myositis, it became immediately evident that I needed to consciously address the question of "what was I willing to do going forward in order to live effectively with this condition?" Without hesitation, my first thoughts centered around my faith in God. Like with everything else in our lives, I knew that I needed His help to move forward effectively. I had always thought of myself as an emotionally strong and stable person. When my mother was dealing with issues associated with her advancing age, and later dementia/Alzheimer's, I prided myself on being there for her. She was always there for me. I was never afraid to take the lead in getting things done in my past...regardless if it was in a personal environment or a work environment. I was always more action-oriented than reaction-oriented.

Julie and I have not been churchgoers over the course of our marriage, nor have we ever been associated with one particular (traditional) religion. Our degree of spirituality and our belief in God was always at a high level, but we came to view our spirituality in conjunction with the ways in which we lived our lives. We believe in the Golden Rule and to treat others in ways that we'd like to be treated ourselves. However, I've always been (and still remain) a huge principles person. By this, I mean that I will stand by my principles. I will not always turn the other cheek when I believe something(s) either goes against my principles or I deem it/them to be inappropriate. I will definitely forgive and move beyond with dignity, but I will not forget.

This inspirational placard is in full view whenever I sit in front of my computer monitor. Julie gave this to me, along with a beautiful cross, after I'd finished my first book. This cross also features the word "hope" and it prominently stands at the right side of this monitor.

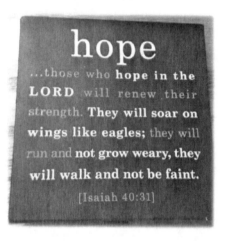

With the passing of time, I've experienced a major change in my relationship with God. It's not only become much more internalized but it's also truly become a more evident part of me. My relationship with God has become consciously omnipresent. Incredibly, it feels like his inspiration has taken over my life and helps me better express who I've become and who I prefer to be. During my book-related presentations, I regularly say that there is absolutely nothing special about me. What's special is that I feel more at peace than I've ever felt before. It's not that I was ever burdened with irreconcilable issues, but I'm now living my life in a way which is highly compatible with where I've advanced spiritually. The phrase, "the peace that passeth all understanding" seems to best describe what's consistently present in my innermost thoughts.

"Praise God, from whom all blessings flow."[25]

---

25 Partial lyrics from a doxology in widespread use in English, in some Protestant traditions commonly referred to simply as "The Doxology" or "The Common Doxology," begins "Praise God, from whom all blessings flow." These words were written in 1674 by Thomas Ken as the final verse of two hymns: "Awake, my soul, and with the sun" and "Glory to thee, my God, this night," intended for morning and evening worship at Winchester College. From Wikipedia, the free encyclopedia.

27

Maintain an Attitude of Gratitude

INITIALLY, WE SELDOM view the various issues and circumstances in our lives in a relative concept. The immediacy of their occurrence has a lot to do with this. When we have some time to think about them, we realize that things could typically be worse. They don't look as bad when we compare them to the alternative(s).

How about if you're given a health diagnosis where you're told, in no uncertain terms, that you have a progressively debilitating disease which has no known treatment or cure...or something similar to this fact? As time passes, should we look at it in relative or absolute terms?

I believe we are most prone to look at things in absolute terms because we take them so personal. If they happen directly or indirectly to us, we find ourselves feeling sorry for ourselves and sometimes even resentful. Now, why did this happen to me?

We are regularly told when we are young to count our blessings. We hear what's been said, but it's easy for someone else to say this when they're not the one being impacted by what is taking place. "If this were to happen to you, you'd feel differently." It's easy to be grateful for things when they're perceived by us as good things.

The dichotomy is why should we be grateful for anything we perceive as bad? My goodness! Acknowledging that we are grateful for bad things in our lives goes against any common sense logic. In absolute terms, this is correct; in relative terms, it is not.

When I was first diagnosed with inclusion body myositis, I honestly did not ask, "Why me?" Yes, I was pretty devastated because in the prior couple of weeks, I had first learned about this disease and what its primary symptoms were. My wife and I realized that I was experiencing some of these symptoms. Did this mean that I was expecting this diagnosis? No, it meant that I recognized that it was a possibility.

The confirmation of this disease hit me square in the face. It was like a bulldozer or a sand truck carrying twenty-six tons of sand. Please see the first chapter of my first book entitled *You Must Answer This* to learn more about this specific reference. The diagnostic call came on a mid-Friday afternoon. I quickly drew on my faith. My goal by Monday morning was to get my head in the right place in order to best deal with this.

There was no intention of wallowing in the aftermath of this disquieting confirmation. That wouldn't do anybody close to me any good, let alone myself. There was really only one option to select from. The other two choices were basically invisible to me. I'd never lived my life this way before, and I was not going to start now. *Such a prognosis is intimidating, but the recipient needs to recognize that there is hope.*

"Some people see things as they are and say why? I dream things that never were and say why not?"[26] (This is a hybrid of an original quote that is credited to author George Bernard Shaw. It was used by and commonly attributed to former United States senator and presidential candidate Robert F. Kennedy)

I find myself consciously counting my blessings. Not that I need any reassurance of them, but when I regularly take some time to identify them…I quickly, and decidedly, realize that I have so much to be grateful for. Yes, things could always be worse. I proudly sat for an interview with a local newspaper reporter not long after my first book was printed. I definitely made the point that if a person dealing with a serious health condition consciously looks around, for only about five seconds, they'll likely identify someone who has it worse off than them.

---

26 Original quote "You see things; and you say "Why?" But I dream things that never were; and I say "Why not?" GEORGE BERNARD SHAW, *Back to Methuselah*, act I, *Selected Plays with Prefaces*, vol. 2, p. 7 (1949). The serpent says these words to Eve.

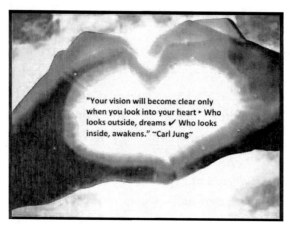

"Your vision will become clear only when you look into your heart ► Who looks outside, dreams ✔ Who looks inside, awakens." ~Carl Jung~

Twin Flame Sacred Keys by Liora (www.twinflame1111.com)

I usually don't attempt to categorize my blessings in relative terms, but there is one exception. My wife, Julie, is truly a major godsend in my life. She is definitely my greatest blessing among many other wonderful blessings.

> She's got a way about her
> I don't know what it is, but I know that I can't live without her She's got a way of pleasin'
> I don't know why it is, but there doesn't have to be a reason anyway She's got a smile that heals me
> I don't know why it is, but I have to laugh when she reveals me And she's got a way of talkin'
> Don't know why it is, but it lifts me up when we are walkin' anywhere She comes to me when I'm feelin' down, inspires me without a sound She touches me and I get turned around"[27]

---

27 Partial lyrics taken from the song "She's Got a Way" written by American singer-songwriter Billy Joel. This was originally

It can be easy, at different times, to get a bit down. It's okay to cry once in a while and get a little upset. It's acceptable to even get mad from time to time. The most important thing, however, is that you have to come back to a better place in a reasonable time frame. That time frame cannot typically be a very long one. Staying in the depths of sorrow or self-pity is not the alternative to choose. We all have different things which make us happy or trip our trigger, so to speak. We need to be conscious of those things. It doesn't matter if it's listening to music, talking with friends, watching a sporting event, reading a book, taking a walk, or simply watching some birds outside a window. There is no greater emotion in our lives than joy. Being in love brings you joy as do many other things. Find them for yourself, because nobody else truly can.

> You must find, and regularly
> utilize, what brings you joy.
>
> —Gary Beyer

released on his first solo album, *Cold Spring Harbor*. It was also featured as a single from the 1981 live album *Songs in the Attic*. en.wikipedia.org.

28

I'm Taking You to Emergency

WE ALL HAVE a tendency to fall into our various routines. The nature of these routines varies over our lifetime. How about our perception of their importance? We sometimes find ourselves out of sorts because a circumstance or unusual matter causes us to deviate from a routine. What if we forget to do something within our normal routine? Heaven forbid!

Most of us are creatures of habit. In fact, I think we're all creatures of habit...if we're allowed to be. I add this important disclaimer because the less independent we become, the more our habits are determinable by others. At the very least, the more influenced they are by our surroundings and personal limitations.

We have our comfort zones too, don't we? "I'm not going to lunch right now, it's too early" or "we should have went to lunch earlier, I'm not even hungry any more." "I'm not wearing this tie to their wedding…I would stand out like a sore thumb." "I'll go there, but I refuse to drive over that higher bridge along the way." "There is no way I'm going to a doctor for this reason. It will heal on its own."

I believe no one truly likes to go to doctors. Periodic, routine visits aren't so bad. Also, if we're being bothered by some specific ailment or readily addressable issue, we're normally thankful to get to a doctor. It's because we believe, after their help and advice, that we'll be feeling better soon. When we're contemplating visiting a doctor because we're unsure of what's going on with us, we're more reluctant to go, but likely recognize that we probably need to.

As a child, I was more bothered by doctor's visits than I've been since that time. I had an ulcer the size of a quarter when I was very young. Drinking the chalky tasting liquid was never that much fun. During first-grade recess, I was hit squarely in the forehead by the backswing of a baseball bat. Thankfully, this was not nearly as powerful as its forward-swing would have been. Some kids were playing baseball, without a catcher, the batter was standing at a blind corner of the school building. I was walking toward this corner, not aware that he was there, and I was suddenly knocked out. I dropped down like a rock and was taken to the local hospital. I ended up getting a huge lump in the center of my forehead and still have the indentation to prove it.

I was pretty healthy over the years. The only surgeries I've had were two that were cataract related and two emergency ones related to retinal-detachment issues. Thanks to the progressive strains of the corporate world, I was diagnosed with Graves's disease (or hyperthyroidism) in my forties. I like to refer to this as "cup runneth over" syndrome. My mother used to say "you can't put ten pounds of sugar in a five-pound sack."

Our desire for routine expands over the years. It broadens to a point where it's no longer exclusive to our home life. We appreciate some degree of it in our school life, our work environment, our social life, and our relationships with those who are closest to us.

There is a high degree of rote behavior associated with our various routines. There is a manner of simplicity as well. Like with any good recipe, we do this then we do that and everything should turn out just fine. Are we possibly taking some things for granted? We commonly think, *If we just follow this routine and simply focus on the other things in my life, we should be all right.*

Is it just me or is the pace of life around us moving faster and faster? With the steady progression of this disease, *I've become much more cognizant of the need to consciously slow down. I love this line from Simon and Garfunkel's song entitled "The 59th Street Bridge Song (Feelin' Groovy)":* "Slow down, you move too fast...you got to make the morning last."[28]

---

28 From Simon and Garfunkel's 1966 album entitled *Parsley, Sage, Rosemary and Thyme.*

Julie and I consciously go to lunch at earlier, less busy times or later, at less busy times. When we go to dinner, we prefer to get there earlier than later and leave before it gets too crowded or noisy. We regularly eat our meals at home at less predictable times. We aren't committed to a routine whereby we attempt to eat our daily meals at specific times. You find that life is too short to be as routine-oriented as you once were. There is an exception, however, which applies to the taking of medication and supplements which are best taken in more of a routine manner.

We get accustomed to certain things in our daily lives. Even when the complications associated with various health conditions come into our lives, we find ourselves getting somewhat used to the changes or adaptations we've needed to make because of them. We detect physical changes in our bodies as well as some new emotional considerations in our minds.

Starting in late August/early September of 2014, I started noticing an unusual pain in the upper inner thigh area of my right leg. It was bothersome, but not overly painful. Because of the muscle condition I have, I regularly try to sit in a chair which has an elevated seat. It's best if the seat's height is higher than my knee level, and I've found counter-height chairs to be perfect. Bar stool-height are okay, but if they don't have a footrest, an extended period of dangling my legs can become a bit problematic too.

Julie had scheduled a get-together at a nearby restaurant on September 14th. I knew it was important for me to be there and I planned on going with her. I had been finding that the pain would uncomfortably radiate in an area just below my groin area to above my knee (especially when I was sitting on a stool-like chair). It would keep my attention because it would consistently throb. Initially, I wondered if I had some type of hernia-related complication, but I couldn't think of anything I'd done that could have caused this.

I was contemplating telling Julie that I thought it best if I stayed home because I thought that the extended period of sitting on the stool wouldn't be that tolerable. I went and it wasn't. I kept my mouth shut about it, but I was definitely hurting throughout the time we were there.

Let's fast-forward to eight thirty on Friday evening of September 26th. I was in our bathroom changing into lounge pants. I noticed that the area below my right knee was significantly blown up. When I walked into the living room to show Julie, she quickly said, "What's wrong with you?" I said that I didn't know. She quickly said, "I'm taking you to emergency."

I didn't challenge her comment, but being as late as it was, I thought we could go over to the hospital first thing in the morning. When we got there, the doctor on call proceeded to ask me questions and do a number of tests including blood work. The technician who conducted ultrasound procedures had just left for the evening and was heading back to her home which was about thirty minutes west. Thankfully, they were able to reach her, and she got back as quick as she could. The ultrasound detected a deep vein thrombosis (DVT) or blood clot in the upper area where I was having the pain.

There was a concern for possible cellulitis below the knee as well, and the doctor prescribed an antibiotic known as clindamycin.

A protocol kicked in whereby I was promptly given an abdominal injection of something called Lovenox. Julie was great when asked if she would be able to give me this injection twice per day for the next five days. I would not have been able to do it myself because both of my hands have been significantly impacted by the progression of inclusion body myositis. I wouldn't have been able to procedurally hold the syringe, let alone process the injections. I was also put on a blood thinner right away. We live about five to ten minutes from this hospital and the doctor decided to let me go home. He said if I detected anything unusual that I should promptly get back to the hospital. I was told to make an urgent appointment with my general care practitioner and was able to do so for Monday morning.

Regular appointments were scheduled for INR blood testing (finger pokes) to monitor my blood. I was put on clindamycin for ten days of two tablets three times per day. The pharmacist told Julie some periods of diarrhea could be expected with this. For the ten days I was on it, I experienced no diarrhea. However, later

I started having some significant bowel-related issues. They got progressively worse. It reached a point where I'd have some terrible gas pains and my bowel habits became very weird and extremely impactful in my daily living. I was literally afraid to go anywhere or make any commitments. There became minimal predictability and, at times, there was a good deal of discomfort. I've become extremely limited in what types of toilet arrangements I can utilize anyway.

I had been scheduled to have a colonoscopy near the end of October. I called the gastroenterologist to ask some questions and likely have the colonoscopy rescheduled. I could not get answers or suggestions as to what might have been going on. My father died of colon cancer, so this got very distressing. *This was honestly one of the scariest periods in my entire life.* Thankfully, I had an appointment coming up with my highly respected homeopath who I now see about every six months. She was extremely upset! First, she couldn't believe that I wasn't at least kept overnight at the hospital when it was first detected that I had a DVT; specifically because of its severity and location. Second, she said that the clindamycin should never have been prescribed for me and that it had significantly disrupted my gastrointestinal tract. Third, she said the scary bloodlike particulate I was regularly finding in my bowel movements was clotting material. She said that the associated clotting material was not just coming from the area of the defined clot. She also said that I was very lucky to be alive. The location of the clot was very unusual and ominous.

I was later told by my rheumatologist in January that he was very concerned about the cause of the clot. He strongly recommended that I have an abdominal CT scan before going off the blood thinner. Like my homeopath, he said there was definite cause for concern because the location of the clot was highly unusual. He told me that there could be some type of mass that was precluding the clot. Thankfully, this was not found to be the case. I was to be on the blood thinner with regular INR testing for a six-month period.

Thank God for Julie's expeditious reactions on that night of September 26, 2014. I do not believe in coincidences. I was meant to show her the blown-up lower right leg at that time. The potential outcome could have been the loss of my life. If the clot was to have moved from its location, it could have quickly caused a pulmonary embolism. My endocrinologist also told me that if I had been simply doing some light exercising activity, I could have quickly just collapsed to the floor, dead, for no apparent reason.

There are a couple of important lessons here: First, don't put off until tomorrow what you can do today. Second, listen to your body and heed it's warnings.

29

The Quiet Times and the Regular Refueling Episodes

I'VE LEARNED A lot more about myself since being diagnosed with this rare, untreatable muscle disease at the beginning of 2008. I've also learned a lot more about other people in my life. Over the years, we find ourselves becoming more and more comfortable in our beliefs and in our surroundings. This is very important because it generates a sense of stability within us.

Then if something "rocks your world," as this type of condition does, it causes one to take closer looks at many different things that you simply didn't delve that far into before. It's interesting how our views change when we clear away some clutter that was, at least partially, influencing our interpretations. There's been an unobvious, favorable by-product which has evolved since I was first confronted with the associated prognosis. It has caused me to go further within myself than I ever had gone before and it's provided me with greater clarity on what is truly important in my life. I wouldn't recommend this route to anyone, however.

I sincerely appreciate all the encouragement and support which I receive. It honestly means more to me than I can adequately express in words. Thank God for Julie and the handful of friends who have shown me something extremely incredible. Their selflessness in meaningfully reaching out to me just stands out so much. It continues to help me a great deal!

It's also become more evident to me that we truly spend a great deal of time alone with our thoughts. This time has increased because my mobility and participation in various activities has become more limited because of this pervasive type of disability. There's no getting away from it. For example, the time allotted for sleeping doesn't mean that only sleeping is involved. We wake up for different reasons, but we don't necessarily go right back to sleep. We process and sift different things through our mind. My goodness! Our brain should be at rest at this time, shouldn't it?

My resolve is being consistently challenged in ways that I never could have imagined. I'm a fighter, not a complainer. I do not take this matter lightly. Strange changes are regularly taking place in my life, but I will not run from them.

> Turn and face the strain Ch-ch-changes
> Don't want to be a richer man Ch-ch-ch-ch-changes
> Turn and face the strain Ch-ch-changes
> Just gonna have to be a different man Time may change me
> But I can't trace time[29]

My faith in God is extremely strong. My personal relationship with Him has become more pronounced and my confidence in Him has grown implicitly. There is definitely no misinterpretation here on my behalf. I pray to Him every night and have focused conversations with Him at different times during the day and night.

As I've said, I've never been a "down" person. I'm certainly not starting now. There are times, however, when I recognize that I need some refueling. Some of these times I even feel a bit overwhelmed. I realize, however, that *I need to come back to positivity as quickly as possible*. I can control this. I consciously call on my internal resolve to do so. I think about other important people in my life who have faced an adversity. Even when they didn't overcome it, they fought the good fight with dignity and class.

---

29 "Changes" is a song written by David Bowie, originally released on the album *Hunky Dory* in December 1971 and as a single in January 1972. en.wikipedia.org—Text under CC-BY-SA license.

I've found the most difficult periods can be after we've gone to bed (or in my case, after I've extended the back of my hydraulic lift chair). The most difficult of them is when you're having trouble sleeping during a night and you hear the clock strike at various hours during that same night. This can play with your head, but you need to find ways to overcome it. The first thing I've found is not to attempt to try to fight it, but rather embrace it. Don't beat yourself up because you're experiencing a particularly challenging night. I find myself sitting up for awhile and just thinking through some things or watching TV for a bit.

The hustle-bustle that I once experienced in my life was much more artificial that I realized at the time. It was what you did, right? There were always time deadlines in my past and everything seemed to center around them. The same types of things had to get done repeatedly. As a corporate accountant, I was subject to prescribed closing periods every four to five weeks. The hustle-bustle is, thankfully, gone now. Refueling is now done for a totally different reason. There were refueling episodes before, but they were more compartmentalized. The ones that are in my life now are much more quiet in nature.

There is a heavy emotional burden associated with this type of condition. I consciously try to keep it inapparent to most others. I've found that this is best addressed at night, but infrequently this is not the case. I've learned that this consistently designated quiet time can be so precious for dealing with emotional trauma and other issues that are determinably complex.

When my brother, Doug, was experiencing his array of health difficulties and other complex challenges, he would regularly tell my sister-in-law, "You can't let things overwhelm you." Boy, was he right! You can't let things overwhelm you. They'll try to, but you need to stand up to them. Fortunately, there are many different ways to do so. It doesn't matter if they're health-related, job-related, or family-related. The power of the human mind combined with the grace of the Almighty God is a formidable obstacle for any challenge we may face in our lives. Most importantly, it's up to each of us to recognize this fact and to be sure that both these factors are the primary components in our line of defense.

The most important phrase that I've now incorporated as a part of my everyday life is "not necessarily."

> Having IBM (Inclusion Body Myositis) means coming to grips with a constantly changing life. The perpetual curtailment of activities requires that you rise above the plight. You need to constantly reinvent yourself in order to adapt to yet another limitation and, at the same time, acknowledge the grieving process that comes with these changes. It means learning to let go and yet go on with your life.
> (Dagmar Slaven, fellow IBM sufferer [she's become a friend and is truly a wonderful inspiration to me])

> It's important that we do our best to see things as they are and not what they may appear to be.
> —Gary Beyer

When The Moon Is Shining

Have you ever taken some time to think?

About the interesting places you can go to when the moon shines?

Mind you, I'm not referring to physically traveling anywhere

It's because these invaluable trips only exist within each of our minds

Fortunately, you won't even need to leave your seat or your bed

During such times the costs of the trips are free, but we must travel them alone

They bring these wonderful opportunities to search within ourselves

As we quietly contemplate our intentions to best function with a positive tone

These trips can be both captivating and undeniably disconcerting

The paths we follow will commonly differ and the landing spots will vary

What's most important, however, is that we utilize them as a type of therapy

Because they can be an important resource which shouldn't make us wary

We know our minds can play some tricks on us from
time to time
And overcoming many of our challenges requires
fortitude, faith and hope
Our complete arsenal of available weapons must be
clearly identified
As we shouldn't disregard utilizing various things which
help us cope

—Gary Beyer (4/7/16)

30

My Divinely Inspired Journey

ONE EARLY MORNING in late July of 2013, I was extremely blessed to experience the most incredible "aha moment" in my life. I'll never forget it! It's like it was yesterday. This is saying a lot too, because I was sixty years old at the time and had experienced a good number of memorable moments in my past.

I had just awakened and immediately, *a very strong and clear thought came to my mind.* It decisively prompted me to pursue the writing of a book. The definitive title for this book came to me within only a couple of seconds thereafter. This was unwittingly the beginning of something which has become *So Much Bigger Than Me.*

I found myself divinely inspired to write the book entitled *You Must Answer This.* In the process of doing so,

I found myself to be spiritually driven to such a degree that it still hasn't remotely backed off. The various trials and tribulations associated with this advancing condition have caused Julie and I to become more deliberate in our behavior than we've ever been before. The word "spontaneity" is no longer a part of our vocabulary.

In conjunction with this unanticipated assortment of efforts, I have honestly become much closer to God. It's hard for me to fully explain, but God has definitely become a larger part of me than he had been prior to this. I've realized an epiphany of sorts where God is now truly omnipresent in every aspect of my life. Even though I've not been an attendee of any church for a very long time, my faith in Him was still very strong and our personal relationship was always very important to me. I definitely respect people who regularly attend a church. My spirituality is such that I've never felt the necessity or desire to be a member of any particular church or religion. This is in no way intended to conflict with other people's need to worship God in a more traditional manner.

What has happened since I began writing my first book has been nothing short of incredible. The feedback I was consistently given from the associated true stories I'd e-mail to different people was highly motivational.

Thanks to my friends, John and Rick, this book came alive very quickly. When I think back, the hand of God was definitely ensuring that this was to take place when it did. The likelihood of things coming together as they have, and then strongly continuing on to this day, would be way beyond my level of comprehension if not for my level of faith in God.

In late 2013 and very early 2014, I initiated the process of introducing the completed book to people I already knew by scheduling presentations at five different area restaurants. These were intended to basically be dry runs, but there were nice postings put up in each of them. Not surprisingly, the only people who attended were those who already knew me, but I was totally honored by their attendance. I was given great feedback by each of them. My presentations since that time have become much more polished.

I was proudly interviewed by a local newspaper reporter and an associated story was placed in two of our area papers in February of 2014. This was really a needed catalyst. It provided some invaluable exposure for *You Must Answer This*. A major point I made during this interview was that if we feel too sorry for ourselves, we simply need to look around. In about five seconds, we'll find someone who is worse off than we are. This is so true! Even when we're attempting to deal with some very difficult things, we usually find it could always be worse.

Hi Gary: (6/8/14)

Blessings to you and Julie, for being out there and encouraging others to have hope!!
Please say a prayer for my brother-in-law. He will be have surgery tomorrow morning at Univ.

of WI hospital in Madison, for a really rare skin cancer (only 300 people in the world have this), which will result in him losing his eye (tumor behind the eyeball, spread into bone, but thank God, not his brain).

Good things to both of you guys!!

Marsha (friend)

In a separate e-mail from May 3, 2014, Marsha also wrote,

I TRULY am enjoying (still not done) reading your book!!! Boy YOU WON THE LOTTERY WITH JULIE!

I couldn't agree with her more.

I was very humbled and honored to be the guest of Fox news reporter Robert Hornacek on his Sunday morning special interest TV show called *Focus*. This interview provided some important validation for me and where I was coming from. A video of this show can be found in the media portion of my website www. youmustanswerthis.com. Five minutes after this show aired, I received a call from a gentleman named Larry who was diagnosed with IBM the previous October. He was able to watch most of the show and was able to find my telephone number. I told him that I'd like to meet with him. The next day, I was able to visit with both he and his wife for quite some time at a local restaurant. They were upbeat people, but he thought he'd been given a death sentence. He told me that he'd recently updated his will because of this. It was obvious that they appreciated my input, as well as the time we were able to spend together. Fox's CW14 actually reaired this show two more times. Shortly after the first airing, I also received a nice e-mail from a lady in Cork, Ireland, who wanted to buy a copy of my book for her father-in-law. He was also suffering from IBM. As you know by now, I no longer believe in coincidences!

Hi Gary, (3/20/14)

Nice picture!!! I taped the show on the 9th because I was out of town for the weekend. I watched it when I got home and thoroughly enjoyed it. You did a really good job throughout the whole interview. I saved the tape so I could let my daughter Debbie enjoy it also. I haven't seen her yet to give it to her!

I haven't had the chance to watch the video on IBM yet but plan on watching it soon.

Sorry to hear about your fall and hope you are healing from the injuries you sustained from that. It is not easy to cope with an illness but you are always so positive about everything going on that you are such an inspiration to all of us!

Thanks for keeping me updated.

Correen (friend and former coworker)

Julie has seen the level of blessings which are being manifested in our lives, thanks to my pursuing the writing of *You Must Answer This*. There was never any indecisiveness. It's been full speed ahead. I humbly refer to this as my divinely inspired journey...because I know that this is *exactly what this is*. I sincerely take no credit for any of the wonderful things that have happened to me since this journey has begun. I've met some outstanding people because of this.

I still remember many of their faces and their first names. I distinctly remember many of their very touching comments. I humbly noticed their facial expressions and body languages as they reacted to my presentations.

I feel as driven as ever to continue giving inspirational presentations. I've given them *at/to libraries, care facilities and nursing homes, seniors' centers, church senior, bereavement and spirituality groups, various support groups (including Parkinson's, cancer survivors, and MDA), colleges, and numerous community organizations.* From March 6 through December 17, 2014, I was able to give a total of fifty presentations throughout this general area of Wisconsin. I'm consistently told that others will benefit from hearing what I have to say. I've been told that I'm a dynamic, motivational speaker. People who are able to attend one of my presentations commonly tell me they are very glad they did. Word has apparently gotten around, because I'm being contacted by people I have never talked with before regarding their interest in having me give a presentation to their respective groups.

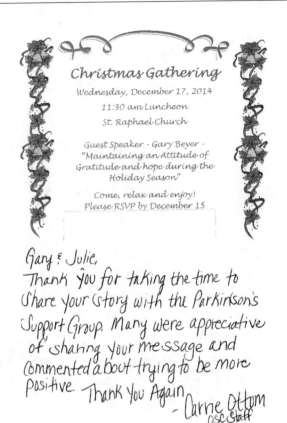

Christmas Gathering

Wednesday, December 17, 2014

11:30 am Luncheon

St. Raphael Church

Guest Speaker - Gary Beyer -
"Maintaining an Attitude of
Gratitude and hope during the
Holiday Season"

Come, relax and enjoy!
Please RSVP by December 15

Gary & Julie,
Thank you for taking the time to share your story with the Parkinson's Support Group. Many were appreciative of sharing your message and commented about trying to be more positive. Thank You Again
  - Carrie Ottom
   OSC Staff

The notice to the left was associated with my fiftieth presentation since March 6, 2014.

There have been some wonderful surprise guests at the various presentations that I have done. I've been extremely moved by this fact. Here are just a handful of examples:

- Our long-time friends, Tim and Diane, showed up at my presentation at the Kimberly Public

Library. We were not expecting them, and it really meant a lot to both Julie and myself. I later had the pleasure of doing a presentation at the care facility where Tim's mother lives. I sure enjoyed visiting with her again.

- The professor of my first accounting class in college was at the presentation I did at the Oshkosh Public Library. I always had a lot of respect for him. It drew some heartfelt tears when I first saw him there. We later taught different sections of a class together. It's still hard calling him Harry instead of Dr. O_____.

- I was totally caught off guard before one presentation when a former coworker arrived in his wheelchair. I always had a lot of respect for George. He has been overcoming a major brain trauma-related issue since I first met him many years ago. He seemed as glad to see me as I was to see him.

- The long-time administrative secretary to the president of a company I'd worked for in my past told me she made it a point to be at a presentation I did to a church group. It really touched me to see Barb and have the opportunity to visit with her before it was to start.

- One of the ladies who used to work directly for me, named Doris, has made it a point to attend two of my presentations (including my very first dry run at our local Perkins Restaurant). She's been just plain classy.

- I was extremely delighted when a former coworker, who I always thought a great deal of, named LaVonne reached out to me. She wanted to attend one of my presentations. We hadn't seen each other for a number of years. She has now attended two of them.
- I was absolutely tickled to see one of my aunt Phyllis's best friends, named Helen, show up at my presentation at our local library. She has subsequently attended two more of my presentations.

In addition to some surprise guests, I've had the opportunity to meet and talk with some very special people I hadn't met previously. Here are just a few examples: (I still can remember the first names of a number of them... so many of them touched me very deeply.)

- I met an eighty-six-year-old gentleman named Reinhold at one of the care facilities I spoke at. He was a Holocaust survivor. After my presentation, he loudly said to the person who I'd first talked with about speaking there, "Where did you find him? You definitely hit a home run this time." I spent about twenty minutes in his room afterward. I'll never forget him...he was extremely interesting!

- Another lady who had cerebral palsy was in a wheelchair in the front row of one of my presentations. Her name was Trish. Her twenty-year-old son was there, as well as her mother and father. She had wanted to write a book. I was proud to visit with her and encourage her.
- We had the pleasure of meeting Jeff and his wife Debbie at another library presentation. Talk about nice people. We really hit it off and have since become friends. He is the head of their book club and has written a couple of books himself. He's also an accomplished musician and has released an impressive CD. There also was another gentleman there named Tom who I also thoroughly enjoyed talking with.
- I also met a lady named Althea at one of the care facilities who really stands out in my mind. She said she'd listened to numerous speakers there, but that I was definitely the best.
- I had the pleasure of meeting and talking with a wonderful lady whose name is Kathy. This was at the same presentation when a fellow myositis warrior named Gail was also gracious enough to be in attendance. She introduced me to Kathy, who told me she lost her husband to IBM a couple of years ago.

We truly enjoyed your presentation yesterday. Lots of positive comments from those I helped back to their rooms. I think it helps them to know that others are also struggling with issues of their own. They realize they are not alone in this "fight." I wish you well on your continued journey of inspiring and uplifting, as well as finding more positives about your illness. Attitude is so important when dealing with anything!! Thank you for your words of encouragement!

Amy (4/1/14)—Life Enrichment Coordinator (for an assisted living and rehabilitation care facility)

Hey Gary! (5/13/14)

It was great to see you present last week. It got me thinking though, and I am wondering if you would be able to switch your date with us one more time. I felt that your message was incredible, and I kept getting this theme of being thankful. With that in mind I was wondering if you would be available to speak at 11:30 a.m. on November 25, 2014 (which should be a Tuesday)?

I hope you are having a wonderful start to your week. I look forward to hearing back from you soon :)

As Always,
Luke (student life assistant/student board advisor/student employment services for a technical college)

Thank you too. You are a delight and upbeat person. I totally agree with everything you said. Since I have been blind all my life, I always hated pity. It isn't pity we need it is understanding. Please tell me the name of your website. I know it is your book title. I hope you sell lots of them. God bless you and Julie.

> Shirley (5/21/14)—(she is a member of a community organization that I spoke to)

Hi Gary, (4/18/14)

Just wanted again to tell you...wonderful job yesterday. I was excited to see you excited.

It is nice to hear how much in love you and Julie are.

Our moms needed to hear what you had to say. Great job. Keep in touch and let me know how you are doing.

Maybe we can hook up down the road.

This job search is not fun, but I have to keep moving. Happy Easter.

> Robin (friend who heard me speak at an assisted living facility)

A wonderful, book-related video was done on *You Must Answer This*. It was thanks to the considerable talents and expertise of Sam. We clicked when we first talked on the telephone, and this was only reinforced when Julie and I met him and his girlfriend soon afterward. He has an uncle who's been suffering from MS. Sam was very understanding and considerate and has become a good friend. This short video can be seen on my website or on YouTube under Youmust answerthis.com.

I'm told that my first book is conversational, enjoyable to read, and quite inspirational to those who've had the opportunity to read it. I believe this one is too. *I Promise I'll Pay Attention* is issues-based, whereas *You Must Answer This* is stories-based. Both books are written from my heart. I believe they're each worth reading. The first book gives the reader reasons to reflect on the multitude of interesting experiences in his/her own life. This second book is insightful for those who are dealing in some way or other with very difficult things in their lives. I'm pleased that I've been able to express what I've wanted to express in each of these books. I am extremely proud of them. The complications from this muscle disease continue to immeasurably affect our lives. Some other significant health-related issues have come into play as well. Regardless of this, my resolve remains steadfast, and I will continue to do my best to help and encourage others.

> It sounds like you are experiencing another round of challenges in your life with your disease. I am grateful we have renewed our friendship because it truly is an inspiration to me to hear how your personal challenges don't hold you back. Gary, I don't mean to sound trite or cliché but God's plan is unfolding in all of this, continue to be an inspiration to people, write, speak, don't let anything hold you back, never give up. Every set back in this life is temporary. Our simple acts of kindness can have a rippling effect. Thank goodness also for Julie, a wonderful partner

indeed for you. I look forward to continuing to hear from you. I hope in the future we can see each other face to face again. Take care my friend and God bless.

Your friend,
Steve (We go back to our junior high days. This was e-mailed to me on Saturday morning, April 18, 2015. Steve and his wife Lynne had recently relocated [back] to Arizona from Washington.)

With Julie retiring last June, she's been able to accompany me to most all my presentations and author fairs since that time. I know she worries about me a great deal and I definitely enjoy and appreciate her company. Being a high school English teacher for thirty-four plus years, she also is an excellent speaker. Being my wife and caregiver, she is able to give people an interesting, firsthand insight on what's taken place in our lives since I was diagnosed with inclusion body myositis. Between the unpredictability of Wisconsin's winter weather and my steadily advancing health condition, Julie and I decided it would be best to err on the side of caution. I consciously decided not schedule more presentations during this specific time frame.

Good morning Gary :)

I am so happy for you that this wonderful inspirational book of yours is now touching so many lives and giving hope and encouragement to so many people, I truly found your story very inspirational myself and your positive outlook amazing.

Gin (4/16/15), senior family service counselor at Mausoleum and Memorial (cemetery) Park

Hello Gary and Julie.

Very well done. Yes your journey in life has lead you to this point and your gift to mankind is your love and enthusiasm that you generate. Thank you for your inspiration and friendship.

Weston (6/18/14), friend and former fellow business owner

We're bombarded with violence, negativity, and sensationalism nearly every day of our lives. In addition to this, the vast majority of us are well-meaning, considerate people. We care for the welfare of others and, especially, for those we've come to know. The problem is we're boring when we're compared to the small percentage of people who aren't well meaning and considerate of others. Unfortunately, it's the other stuff that attracts media attention and gets the bulk of exposure.

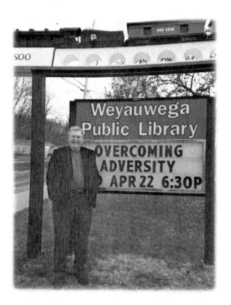

I consistently find myself feeling highly energized and emotionally engaged in these efforts. God willing, I will be able to continue to bring some positive insight and encouragement to those I am able to touch. I sincerely believe that my purpose, the rest of my life, is to help other people be hopeful and encouraged.

—Gary Beyer

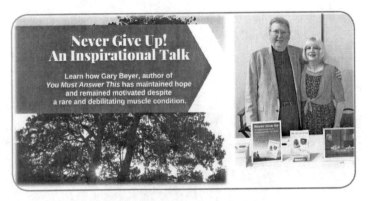

Gary and Julie at Authors Showcase 2015

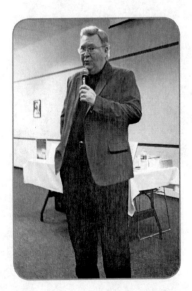

Gary during a presentation at his hometown library in 2015

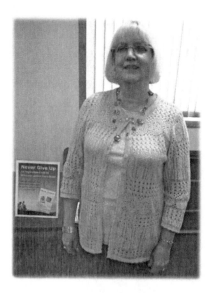

Julie before a presentation

In Closing

You could've, but you chose not to.
You would've, but you didn't.
You should've, but you decided against it.

—Gary Beyer

THERE'S NO GOOD reason to ever let ourselves spend too much of our precious time on regret. It truly is wasted energy that gets us nowhere and resolves absolutely nothing. We make conscious decisions using the best information we have at the time that we make them.

This point does not alleviate the fact that it is our responsibility to make the best decisions possible at the time they are made. We typically make our best decisions when we are proactive and truly engaged in our lives. We are not just acting as a participant, but we are the featured performer.

Be the featured performer. This isn't arrogance, it is cognizance! Be the catalyst for bringing (and keeping) happiness into your lives. This is something you can do.

It really is something you must do…not something you could've, would've, or should've done. We each need to take charge of our lives to the best of our abilities. Health-related issues and other complications can legitimately limit our abilities, but they can't limit our attitudes because we control them as well.

Also, our faith in God needs to be at the forefront of how we live our lives.

"With respect to living with a progressively debilitating disease, I believe it's vitally important to continue to *fight the good fight* while placing your trust in God" (Gary Beyer).

> Keep up your spirit, keep up your faith, baby I am
> counting on you
> You know what you've got to do
> Fight the good fight every moment
> Every minute every day
> Fight the good fight every moment
> It's your only way

Partial lyrics from the song entitled "Fight the Good Fight" (written by Mike Levine, Gil Moore and Rik Emmett of the Canadian rock band Triumph. It's from their *Allied Forces* album which was released in 1981.)

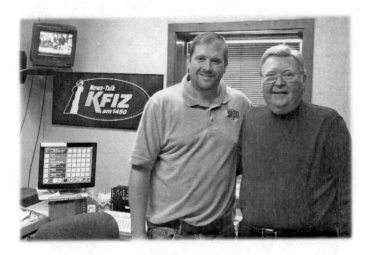

Gary after his KFIZ radio station interview
with program director Wade Bates

Two Specific Reasons for Encouragement

IN THE PAST five years, more positive developments have taken place in the way of medical research than have occurred in the prior fifty years. This is not only exciting. It represents life-changing encouragement for many people who are doing their best to deal with life-altering diseases and conditions every day of their lives!

Sporadic inclusion body myositis (sIBM) continues to be a major stumper in the world of medical research, but I believe that significant progress is finally being made. The complexity of this disease has inevitably caused failed efforts up to this point. Thankfully, the conviction associated with such efforts has not been exhausted. There is no intended conjecture as to the eventual level of success to be realized from either of the following two efforts. The important thing is that they are both in the works and they each carry reasons for encouragement.

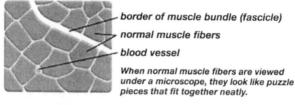

border of muscle bundle (fascicle)

normal muscle fibers

blood vessel

When normal muscle fibers are viewed under a microscope, they look like puzzle pieces that fit together neatly.

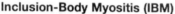

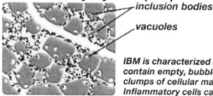

inclusion bodies

vacuoles

IBM is characterized by muscle fibers that contain empty, bubble-like spaces (vacuoles) and clumps of cellular material (inclusion bodies). Inflammatory cells can be seen between the fibers.

New compound could reverse loss of muscle mass

A new antibody could dramatically boost strength and muscle mass in patients with cancer, chronic obstructive pulmonary disease (COPD), sporadic inclusion body myositis, and in elderly patients with sarcopenia.

This new research was published in the journal *Molecular and Cellular Biology* (2013; doi:10.1128/MCB.01307-13).

"Age-related loss of muscle mass is a major contributing factor to falls, broken bones, and the loss of mobility," said co-corresponding author David Glass, MD, of Novartis, in Cambridge, Massachusetts, one of the compound's developers, along with first author Dr. Estelle Trifilieff, also of Novartis. "This study illustrates that we may have a powerful tool to prevent muscle wasting and promote growth."

The new compound (BYM338) acts to prevent muscle wasting by blocking a receptor that engages a cellular signaling system that exists to put the brakes on muscle development when appropriate. But sometimes those brakes are activated inappropriately, or become stuck.

"Our goal was to release the brakes," said Glass.

A variety of signals can activate the receptor. Prior to development of BYM338, compounds developed to block these molecules were blunt instruments, either trapping all incoming signals (which stimulated muscle growth but also caused harmful side effects) or blocking just a single receptor activator (providing only tepid growth stimulation). BYM338 was designed to be in the Goldilocks zone (just right).

In the study, the compound boosted muscle mass 25% to 50%, and increased strength in animal models. Those gains were significantly superior to those of compounds that blocked a single receptor activator. Clinical trials are currently underway.

The condition that BYM338 is designed to treat is loss of skeletal muscle and fat, which is not reversed by simply eating more, and is known as cachexia when associated with certain chronic illnesses. Cancer cachexia develops in a majority of patients with advanced malignancy, and can interfere with the ability to undergo chemotherapy, said Glass. COPD afflicts an estimated 65 million people worldwide and is predicted to become the third leading cause of death by 2020. As many as a quarter of COPD patients suffer from cachexia, which can worsen already dire respiratory difficulties.

Sarcopenia—age-related loss of muscle and physical function—afflicts 5% to 13% of persons age 60 to 70 years, rising to 11% to 50% in persons older than 80 years. These people become especially vulnerable to falling. Among older adults, falls are the leading cause of both fatal and nonfatal injuries, according to the Centers for Disease Control and Prevention.

Preliminary data on the antibody was promising enough to have it designated as a breakthrough therapy by the US Food and Drug Administration for sporadic inclusion body myositis, a rare muscle wasting disease with no approved therapies.

"We need to be able to help people maintain productive and meaningful lives, and muscle function is a major part of the equation," said Glass. "It could be the difference between independent living and having to move into a nursing home."

Oncology Nurse Advisor January 15, 2014

(Kathy Boltz, PhD)

Only nine days after I started writing my first book, *You Must Answer This*, I received an e-mail from friend and fellow myositis warrior, Jim Szudzik, letting me know of something very special which had just taken place. This information immediately follows: (As you know, I don't believe in coincidences!)

Media Releases

August 20, 2013 07:15 CET

Novartis receives FDA breakthrough therapy designation for BYM338 (bimagrumab) for sporadic inclusion body myositis (sIBM)

- Designation highlights potential of BYM338 to address an unmet medical need in a serious disease
- If approved, BYM338 has the potential to be the first treatment for sIBM patients
- BYM338 is the third Novartis investigational treatment this year to receive a breakthrough therapy designation by the FDA, highlighting Novartis's leadership in the industry in breakthrough therapy designations Basel, August 20, 2013—Novartis announced today that the US FDA has granted breakthrough therapy designation to BYM338 for sIBM.

Breakthrough therapy designation was created by the FDA to expedite the development and review of new drugs for serious or life-threatening conditions. This designation is based on the results of a phase II proof-of-concept study that showed BYM338 substantially benefited patients with sIBM compared to placebo. The results of this study will be presented at the American Neurological Association meeting on October 14 and is expected to be published in a major medical journal later this year.

sIBM is a rare yet potentially life-threatening, muscle-wasting condition. Patients who have the disease can gradually lose the ability to walk, experience falls, and injuries, lose hand function, and have swallowing difficulties[30]. There are no currently approved (or established) treatment options for sIBM[31].

"BYM338 is the third example this year of Novartis's leadership in bringing breakthrough therapies to patients reinforcing our commitment to innovation addressing significant unmet medical needs and enhancing the lives of patients," said Timothy Wright, MD, global head of development, Novartis Pharmaceuticals. "With no effective therapies currently available for sIBM, bimagrumab has the potential to be the first real option for patients with this condition."

About BYM338 (bimagrumab) and the Novartis commitment to research in muscle therapeutics:

BYM338 (bimagrumab) is a novel, fully human monoclonal antibody developed to treat pathological

---

30 [Note: Provide source.] ClinicalTrials.gov Identifier: NCT01519349

31 [Note: Provide source.] Sponsor: Nationwide Children's Hospital

muscle loss and weakness. BYM338 was developed by the Novartis Institutes for Biomedical Research (NIBR), in collaboration with MorphoSys, whose HuCAL library was used to identify the antibody. BYM338 binds with high affinity to type II activin receptors, preventing natural ligands from binding, including myostatin and activin. BYM338 stimulates muscle growth by blocking signaling from these inhibitory molecules.

In addition to being developed for sIBM, BYM338 is in clinical development for COPD, cancer cachexia, sarcopenia, and in mechanically ventilated patients. BYM338 is administered by intravenous infusion.

"Follistatin Gene Transfer to Patients with Becker Muscular Dystrophy and Sporadic Inclusion Body Myositis"

ClinicalTrials.gov—
A Service of the US National Institutes of Health

Purpose

The investigators are performing a gene therapy clinical trial in Becker muscular dystrophy (BMD) and **sporadic inclusion body myositis (sIBM)** patients. Both of these conditions have an important common feature: loss of ability to walk because of weakness of the thigh muscles. The investigators plan to do a gene therapy trial to deliver a gene to muscle called follistatin (FS344) that can build muscle size and strength.

If successful, the investigators can increase the size of the thigh muscle and potentially prolong a patient's ability to walk. The gene will be carried into the muscle by a virus called adeno-associated virus (AAV). This virus occurs naturally in muscle and does not cause any human disease, setting the stage for its safe use in a clinical trial.

Presently there is no treatment that can reverse Becker muscular dystrophy or sporadic inclusion body myositis. Only supportive care is currently possible.

In this study, subjects with either of these diseases will have shots of the follistatin gene injected directly into thigh muscle on one (first cohort) or both legs (2nd and 3rd cohort). One hundred and eighty days following the gene delivery, the muscle will undergo biopsy to look closely at the muscle to see if the muscle fibers are bigger. Between the time of the gene transfer and the muscle biopsy, patients will be carefully monitored for any side effects of the treatment. This will include an MRI of the thigh muscle before treatment and at day 180 following treatment. Blood and urine tests, as well as physical examination will be done on the subjects during the screening visit and on days 0, 1, 2, 7, 14, 30, 60, 90, and 180 to make sure that there are no side effects from the gene injections. Sutures will be removed 2 weeks post-biopsy.

Additional blood samples will be collected at 9, 12, 18, and 24 months. Patients will be seen at the end of 1st and 2nd years for a physical exam, assessment of muscle strength and appropriate blood tests.

"BMD, IBM: Preliminary Findings in Follistatin Gene Transfer Study Promising"

Early data show follistatin gene transfer may be safe and effective in BMD and safe in IBM, in which efficacy has not yet been evaluated.

BY MARGARET WAHL ON NOVEMBER 7, 2013—3:00PM

Preliminary results from a trial to test the safety of injecting *follistatin* genes into the thigh muscles of adults with **Becker muscular dystrophy (BMD)or sporadic (nongenetic) inclusion-body myositis (sIBM)** suggest that the experimental therapeutic approach is safe in both types of patients, and that it may improve walking ability in BMD. (Efficacy in IBM patients has not yet been evaluated.)

Follistatin is a protein that interferes with the actions of *myostatin*, a protein known to inhibit muscle growth.

Neurologist, Jerry Mendell, the principal investigator on this study, reported the preliminary findings at the 2013 annual meeting of the Child Neurology Society (CNS), held in Austin, Texas, Oct. 30-Nov. 2.

About the follistatin gene transfer study

The follistatin gene transfer study is being conducted at Nationwide Children's Hospital in Columbus, Ohio, where Mendell directs the Center for Gene Therapy and the Paul D. Wellstone Muscular Dystrophy Clinical Research Center, and where he co-directs the MDA neuromuscular disease clinic.

The trial began after animal studies conducted in the laboratory of Brian Kaspar, a research scientist at Nationwide Children's, showed follistatin has therapeutic potential.

Mendell is a longtime MDA research grantee, but this follistatin gene- transfer trial is being funded by Parent Project Muscular Dystrophy (PPMD) and the Myositis Association.

Enrollment of BMD patients is complete. Men with BMD who were ambulatory and met other study criteria received an injection of follistatin genes encased in delivery vehicles derived from *type 1 adeno-associated viruses (AAV1s) into a thigh muscle in both legs.*

Preliminary results in BMD encouraging

Two trial participants with BMD have completed one year of evaluations since receiving low-dose follistatin gene injections. One has increased the distance he is able to walk in six minutes *(six-minute walk distance, or 6MWD)* compared to his baseline 6MWD by 111 meters (364 feet), and the other by 56 meters (184 feet). A third participant with BMD, who has so far been evaluated six months after receiving the low-dose injections, has increased his 6MWD by 13 meters (43 feet).

Mendell also reported that a participant with BMD who received a higher dose of follistatin genes has increased his baseline 6MWD by 54 meters (177 feet) one month after the injections were administered. "We will be continuing to follow him," Mendell said, adding, "I want to stress that this is preliminary data."

There have been no adverse events.

Testing in IBM patients underway

The follistatin gene transfer trial is also designed to include adults with **sporadic (nongenetic) inclusion-body myositis (IBM)**. Mendell noted that three trial participants with IBM received a very low dose of follistatin genes injected into one leg muscle and were evaluated on safety measures alone. IBM-affected participants will now receive doses comparable to those given to participants with BMD. No adverse events have been seen in the IBM patients.

Mendell invites adults with IBM who are able to walk without assistance and want to be screened for possible participation in the follistatin gene- transfer study to email him at Jerry.Mendell@nation widechildrens.org.

This article was reprinted in: *Quest—MDA's Research & Health Magazine*

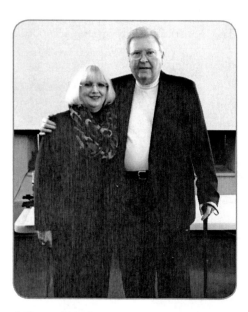

Julie and Gary after their presentation at the West Bend
Community Memorial Library in October of 2015.

The Same Words and Phrases, But They Have Altered Meanings

Achievement
Before: Some type of defined accomplishment.
Now: Getting something done.

Normal
Before: A taken-for-granted circumstance, relationship, or matter.
Now: Nothing is taken for granted, normal is ever-changing.

Weekend
Before: Something we longed for every week of our lives.
Now: Two of the seven other days in a week.

Rainy days and Mondays
Before: Relatively depressing and a regular basis for complaining.
Now: Appreciated, like any other day in our lives.

Rare
Before: Something distinctively uncommon and likely of significant value.
Now: Something distinctively uncommon that you don't want to experience.

Constraints
Before: Limitations which are externally created and outside of our control.
Now: Any limitations which are outside of our control.

Taking a trip
Before: Traveling more than one hundred miles.
Now: Heading to the nearby grocery store or to another destination in town.

Vacation
Before: That one- or two-week getaway from work.
Now: Somewhat confused by what his means.

Climbing the stairs or walking up steps
Before: Not a particularly significant issue.
Now: There's increasing difficulty stepping up on a curb, let alone attempting to climb stairs (this currently cannot be accomplished without the use of my EZ-Step device and a sturdy handrail)

Changing my pants
Before: No issues.
Now: There better be a counter I can put my back against or a wall I can lean against.

Raising my legs
Before: No issues.

Now: Not so fast, my friend…neither of my legs can be raised very far any more.

Visit
Before: Talking face to face for a half hour or more with a friend or acquaintance.
Now: Talking on the telephone for five to ten minutes with anyone.

Using a bathroom
Before: Not an issue, to be used as necessary.
Now: A limited option if I can't get up from the toilet seat without help (most of the toilet setups I just can't use without an assistive feature).

Getting into and out of a vehicle
Before: Not an issue from either the driver's or passenger sides.
Now: This condition has made me so inflexible that I cannot get in or out of numerous vehicles.

Completing a small project
Before: No issues.
Now: Takes longer than one or two days to complete and is not necessarily planned.

Sleeping in a bed
Before: No issues.

Now: My bed has become a hydraulic lift chair, I have great difficulty getting up from a flat surface.

Tickets for a Milwaukee Brewers baseball game
Before: Anywhere in the infield area, but as close to home plate as possible.
Now: An ADA seat in the infield area where I can utilize my director's-height chair.

Comfortable
Before: Anything that felt especially good.
Now: Anything that feels better than it otherwise could.

Swallowing
Before: Something I took for granted with or without food.
Now: Without food, there's some bending down of my chin and with food, there's slower, more deliberate chewing supported with small sips of liquid.

Taking a good walk
Before: Covering close to an hour in time, regardless of distance.
Now: Anything that covers no more than two to three blocks (this is steadily changing).

Preferential treatment
Before: Above and beyond services or assistance.

Now: Not a matter of special treatment, but rather associated with general accessibility

Using a ladder
Before: Not that big of a deal, but being sure to be careful.
Now: No longer an option for me (regardless if it's a small stepladder).

What if I'd fall or be down on the ground
Before: Not that big of a deal, I'd simply get back up.
Now: Couldn't even get myself on a knee for one hundred thousand dollars, let alone get up without paramedic-type help.

Difficult
Before: something challenging and perceived as hard to accomplish.
Now: Anything that seems potentially unable to complete.

Being innovative
Before: Incorporating unobvious ideas and pursuing atypical solutions.
Now: Identifying alternative ways of doing, what most people consider to be, very simple things.

Tying a shoelace
Before: No big deal, didn't think twice about it.
Now: Both difficult and avoided.

Taking a walk in the grass
Before: Thoroughly enjoyed it with no issues.
Now: The normal variability found in a surface makes this a challenging experience.

Watching a desirable, "live" music concert
Before: Enjoying the concert in person, if possible and practical.
Now: Viewing it on a TV screen or from a nicely recorded DVD.

Close friend
Before: A steady companion and confidant, someone you'd trust and enjoy activities with.
Now: A compassionate and considerate confidant, someone who's consistently shown a genuine interest in my well-being.

A bad day
Before: A relatively frustrating day which is filled with problems, bad weather, and/or disturbing news or bother-some things.
Now: This phrase has become less associated with external matters and has become more associated with comparative physical issues and complications experienced from one day to another (there are very few bad days…rather, one day is not quite as good as the prior one was).

Just about supper/dinnertime
Before: Around 6:00 or 6:30 p.m.
Now: Sometime between 5:30 p.m. and 8:00 p.m.

Early in the morning
Before: Around 5:00 a.m.
Now: Any time before 8:00 a.m.

I'm so proud to confirm that this book was initially completed on May 10, 2015. This represents a very special day for me. It is Mother's Day and also would have been my father's 109th birthday.

I've always said that if I could be half the person my father was I'd consider myself successful. I learned from him the most important lesson that I've ever learned in my life. That lesson is to treat other people the way you'd like to be treated yourself.

Father's Day this year is to fall on Sunday, June 21st. I was born on June 21st of 1953... which also happened to be Father's Day that year. This is all very interesting to me as I do not believe in coincidences.

(Gary Beyer)

Personal Testimonies

"I had the real pleasure of attending Gary and Julie Beyer's stellar presentation in the fall of 2015. I was greatly inspired by Gary's uplifting and very positive attitude toward life and the circumstances that he has been dealt. His wife Julie's part of the presentation is a true testament to how important the right caregiver is to a person who is going through such a life-threatening event. Both Gary and Julie in their presentation creatively blended comedy with true life lessons for us all!

"The most important thing I gleaned from their enlightening presentation is that a person's serious illness can have a double whammy effect, as a lot of times close friends start avoiding the person with the illness as they do not know how to act around or what to say to the person or their caregiver. This in turn causes social isolation for the person and their caregiver, and I deeply feel this is the worst part of the illness. We cannot allow this social isolation to continue to happen!"

—Mark R. Weisensel, MSE, APSWSupervisor of Winnebago County Aging and Outreach Services

"Gary, good morning to you. I'm so excited for you about your new book. People do need to realize that none of the situations we find ourselves living in are always going to be easy. Some even constantly test our faith and perseverance! Thank goodness none of us have to go through these experiences alone on our journey through our lifetime. We all need one another as we go along this bumpy road that we travel so that we continue to realize that as people we are often more alike than different in the way that we face our everyday struggles; I strongly feel that this is the only way each of us can, and will, find true *peace* within ourselves as individuals! This is what you, Gary Beyer, have allowed me to find within my heart and soul; the inner peace that I now feel as a result of writing about some very difficult situations in my lifetime. It allowed me to explain how I felt going through some of the situations that I had to go through living with cerebral palsy. Thanks to you and Julie for your friendships. I don't know what I would do without them! I'm so happy for each of you and proud of you both; you really have learned how to persevere in a difficult situation *together*! I am not ashamed of myself anymore! You, my friend, are a true blessing in the form of a human being! Thank you for allowing me this opportunity to be able to further heal from the awful pain and suffering that I have been carrying around for most of my lifetime! Congrats and love always."

—Moonbeam(May 15, 2015 email)